Chicken Soup for the Soul.

Say Goodbye to Back Pain!

D0377669

Chicken Soup for the Soul: Say Goodbye to Back Pain!
How to Handle Flare-Ups, Injuries, and Everyday Back Health
by Dr. Julie Silver

Published by Chicken Soup for the Soul Health, an imprint of Chicken Soup for the Soul Publishing, LLC www.chickensoup.com
Copyright © 2012 by Chicken Soup for the Soul Publishing, LLC. All Rights Reserved.
No part of this publication may be reproduced, stored in a retrieval system or transmitted in any form or by any means, electronic, mechanical, photocopying, recording or otherwise, without the written permission of the publisher.

Chicken Soup for the Soul Health, CSS Health, CSS, Chicken Soup for the Soul, and its Logo and Marks are trademarks of Chicken Soup for the Soul Publishing LLC.

The publisher gratefully acknowledges the many publishers and individuals who granted Chicken Soup for the Soul permission to reprint the cited material.

This publication contains the opinions and ideas of the authors. It is intended to provide helpful and informative material on the subjects addressed in the publication. Harvard Medical School and the publisher are not engaged in rendering medical, health, psychological, or any other kind of personal professional services in the book. The reader should consult a health professional before adopting suggestions in this book.

Harvard Medical School, the authors and the publisher specifically disclaim all responsibility for any liability, loss, or risk, personal or otherwise, incurred as a direct or indirect consequence of the use and application of any of the contents of this book.

Front cover and interior photo courtesy of iStockphoto.com/NadyaPhoto (© Nadya Lukic).
Back cover photo of Dr. Julie Silver courtesy of Kent Dayton.

Cover and Interior Design & Layout by Pneuma Books, LLC
For more info on Pneuma Books, visit www.pneumabooks.com

Distributed to the booktrade by Simon & Schuster. SAN: 200-2442

Publisher's Cataloging-In-Publication Data
(Prepared by The Donohue Group, Inc.)

Silver, J. K. (Julie K.), 1965-

 Chicken soup for the soul : say goodbye to back pain! : how to handle flare-ups, injuries, and everyday back health / Julie Silver.

 p. : ill. ; cm.

 Summary: A collection of stories on the topic of managing back and neck injuries and recovery, including diagnosis, treatment, exercises, and ongoing maintenance of back and neck health, accompanied by medical advice.

 ISBN: 978-1-935096-87-0

 1. Back--Care and hygiene--Popular works. 2. Backache--Popular works. 3. Neck pain--Popular works. 4. Back--Care and hygiene--Anecdotes. 5. Backache--Anecdotes. 6. Neck pain--Anecdotes. I. Title. II. Title: Say goodbye to back pain

PN6071.B25 S55 2012

810.2/02/356/1   2012931532

PRINTED IN THE UNITED STATES OF AMERICA
on acid∞free paper

21 20 19 18 17 16 15 14 13 12   01 02 03 04 05 06 07 08 09 10

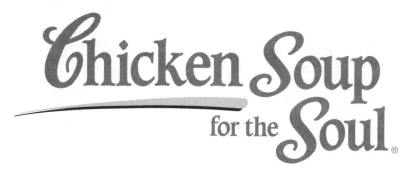

Chicken Soup for the Soul®

Say Goodbye to Back Pain!

How to Handle Flare-Ups, Injuries, and Everyday Back Health

by **DR. JULIE SILVER** of
HARVARD MEDICAL SCHOOL

Chicken Soup for the Soul Publishing, LLC
Cos Cob, CT

Contents

Chapter 4

Chapter 5

Chapter 6

Chapter 7

Chapter 8

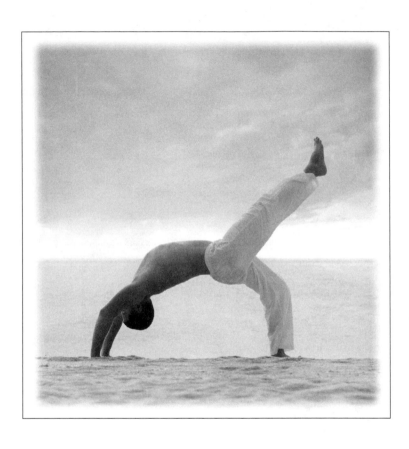

Chapter 1
Oh, My Aching Back!

The Weight of War

I t hurts so bad.

It started the day I was issued my body armor, which weighs 30 to 40 pounds alone. Include the rifle, pistol, additional ammo, water, and other assorted tools that the American soldier wears, and that gear can weigh anywhere from 60 to 100 pounds. Add in the fact that I only weigh 135 pounds and have a weaker-than-normal skeletal frame to begin with, and it's no wonder I didn't last a day before I crumpled to the ground under the weight of my gear.

It was fortunate that this happened at a training event; just a few months later, I'd be in Afghanistan, and collapsing in the middle of a mission would be disastrous. Instead, I was able to lie down until I could regain my strength.

A few days after my collapse, I was given improved armor that distributed the weight better over my whole body. But the damage was already done: my back would never be the same, ranging from bitter pain to utter numbness.

During my time in Afghanistan, my back became progressively worse. I had seen the military doctors a few times, but they weren't able to offer much help other than specific stretches intended to release the tension in my spine and hip.

I woke up on Easter morning in the worst condition I'd ever been in, so I limped over to the Troop Medical Center. Specialist Chris Talbert was the medic in the TMC that day.

"Sergeant, where does it hurt?" he asked.

"I'm feeling pain at the bottom of my back," I tried explaining, "and it shoots through my right hip and down the leg, stopping at the knee, but then striking again just below my ankle. But the ankle itself is numb."

Spc. Talbert nodded his head and noted everything I had told him. It was a textbook case: I had a bulging disc, also known as a herniated disc, also known as a slipped disc, also known as a screwed-up back. By the end of my visit, I was given some painkillers to help me lie down at night.

Three months later, Spc. Talbert was dead. During a mission, his convoy rolled over an anti-tank mine. While several soldiers were there during the explosion, Spc. Talbert was the only one who didn't walk away from the blast.

I survived the rest of my tour in Afghanistan, but I haven't escaped its permanent effects on my body. At night, I'll wake up and cry out in pain as my back will shoot tiny little bullets through my entire body, except for my left leg, which is spared because it is numb. When the pain is especially intense, I'll get out of bed and stretch, just hoping that maybe some of the strain will be alleviated.

Once or twice, I've been tempted to feel sorry for myself. "If it weren't for the Army, I'd be whole!" "Poor me. I'll never be the same again." Or, here's my favorite: "Nobody understands how bad this hurts."

But then I remember those soldiers who lost a lot more than I did. I remember Spc. Talbert who died while assisting others, just as he had assisted me. If at any time I am about to forget his legacy, I just whip out his handwritten medical assessment of my back and I am reminded of the greater sacrifices so many have given. What they would do to feel back pain again!

I still feel sore when I lie down at night. It still wakes me up, and I still cry out in pain. But you know what? If I can feel pain, then it means I'm still alive.

It hurts so good.

— Sgt. Danger Geist —

Back in the Saddle

All my life I wanted a horse. As a little girl, I put every dime I got into the mechanical horse at the grocery store, bouncing down make-believe trails. I counted the days until our annual summer visit to friends with Shetland ponies that took me for rides. Every horse book in the children's library had my name on the checkout card. As an adult, I held onto the dream, hoping some day to ride my very own horse.

To celebrate turning fifty, I bought an Arabian mare the color of a copper penny. Vida, trained well enough for a novice rider, was perfect for me. We spent a few days getting to know each other at the small barn where I boarded her. Then I led her into the arena and, with the coaching of an instructor, saddled up and swung on. Vida stood quietly while I settled onto the saddle, with a huge smile on my face.

By the time we'd circled the arena three times, my smile had turned to a grimace. My back hurt so much I had to rein Vida in and climb off.

True, I wasn't as young as when I'd ridden the mechanical pony. But an aching back after such a short ride? And Vida and I had only walked, not trotted or cantered. My back ached sometimes when I'd been on my feet a long time at work or after fixing dinner for company, but not like this.

I knew women in their fifties and sixties who rode. My idol was an eighty-year-old woman who got on her bicycle every morning and pedaled twenty minutes to a barn where she boarded her horse. Then she brushed and saddled her horse, and rode for half an hour. I wasn't a sedentary person. I walked, biked, and occasionally hiked. Was horseback riding really such a demanding sport? Or was there something seriously wrong with my back?

When I returned Vida to her pasture, she extended her neck for me to stroke the white blaze that ran the length of her nose. "What am I going to do?" I asked, looking into her soft, brown eyes.

She nickered softly. I swear that nicker was "exercise" in horse talk.

I made an appointment with an osteopath who had helped me with a knee injury two years before.

"Where does it hurt?" he asked.

"My mid back and lower back."

As he aligned me with gentle stretches, he reassured me that he felt no arthritis. An X-ray revealed no disc problems. I simply had a weak back, perhaps because all my life I'd had round shoulders and now had mild scoliosis.

"I just bought a horse and I want to ride her," I told him. "It's my dream."

"Work hard," he said as he handed me a prescription for physical therapy.

I didn't mind working hard cleaning Vida's stall, but back exercises sounded boring. However, I read online that a rider needs certain muscles to properly cue a horse. Furthermore, the soundness of a horse's back is affected by the balance and posture of the rider. A weak back would not only hurt me, it would also hurt my beautiful mare. I telephoned the physical therapy office and made an appointment for their first opening.

In physical therapy I learned to make a hip bridge, lying on my back lifting my hips so they made a straight line from hips to shoulders. I did a fair imitation of a bird dog, starting on hands and knees with a neutral back and extending my right leg and left arm, then reversing sides. I lunged across the floor of the therapist's workout room with hands on hips, alternating knees at a ninety-degree angle with my lower legs. I even did a side plank. Lying on my side, I contracted my abs and lifted my hips so there was a straight line from knees to shoulders. Sweat soaked my T-shirt. Did I want to ride this badly? I pictured myself galloping Vida across a field, wildflowers bending beneath her flying hooves. Yes, I did.

Figuring thirteen-year-old Vida could have back issues as well, I learned stretches and exercises that would help strengthen her back and we did them every time I visited the barn.

For two weeks I faithfully did my exercises. I wanted to do more than brush Vida's mane and tail, pick her feet, and lead her around the arena. The day I arrived to ride her again, Vida lifted her head from grazing and whinnied to me. I shivered with excitement. "Hi, girlfriend," I called as I walked toward the fence.

She ambled over and took a carrot from my hand. As I listened to her crunch, I slipped through the gate and wrapped my arms around her neck. "It's going to be different today," I promised.

I tacked up and climbed on, expecting to walk five laps around the arena, then cue Vida into a brisk trot. To my dismay, walking five laps was my limit. How long was I going to need to do my back exercises?

I thought of a biking friend who had injured a hip so badly in a fall that he couldn't bike without first doing a series of stretches. He didn't own a car and biked everywhere, which meant he did the exercises every single day. I breathed out. Would that be my fate?

I confided my struggle to a neighbor. "Yoga's what you need to strengthen your back," she insisted, and handed me a card for a local studio. "Alignment and core stability. Here's where I go. The instructors are all physical therapists."

It did sound like what I needed. I began taking weekly yoga classes and established a home practice that included locust, cobra, downward dog and plank pose. I wondered if any yoga positions were named after horses. As I lay on my yoga mat, lifting my breastbone and pulling my shoulder blades together, I pictured myself sitting tall in Vida's saddle. I had to keep at it.

For another month I brushed Vida's shining copper coat, and put her through a series of stretches. I lounged her, feeding the loops of line as she walked, trotted and cantered around me. I did my physical therapy exercises and yoga home practice daily. My yoga teacher remarked that I was standing straighter.

Six weeks from the day I first rode Vida, I mounted for the third time, patting her lovely arched neck and thanking her for her patience. We walked five laps each direction and trotted two laps before I grew uncomfortable. "Progress," I told her, dismounting and hugging her neck.

Each time I rode, Vida and I went a little further. Delight consumed me every time I got back in the saddle. I knew before long we'd be exploring trails together. Thanks to strong backs—mine and hers—my dream had come true.

~ Samantha Ducloux Waltz ~

Someone to Watch Over Me

"Back surgery is definitely out of the question," I indignantly informed my orthopedic surgeon after his examination in 2003. I painfully informed him of my decision as I was bent at a ridiculous 90-degree angle. Realizing my back was in a preposterous predicament for negotiation, I still demanded other options. After all, I had worked in the health and fitness field for 20 years and my experience as a Health and Fitness Director had exposed me to many serious back injuries. Not one person I knew had come through back surgery better off than before they succumbed to the scalpel.

I did, however, know several people who experienced constant back pain ever since their surgery, including my dad and brother. No sir—I was not ready to "hang up my athletic sneakers" for an extremely painful sedentary life in a rocking chair. I may have needed someone to watch over me, but I was not convinced it would be an orthopedic surgeon.

"I want to know my other options," I entreated the surgeon.

"Your only other option..." the expert said in a non negotiating tone, "is a life of agonizing pain bound to a wheelchair."

Now he had my full attention. I timidly inquired, "When do you think I should have surgery if I decide on that option?" I was really hoping to put off surgery indefinitely on the outside chance my back would heal itself.

"I am leaving the country in two weeks to visit my family in Ireland. I will be gone a month. I don't think you will be able to tolerate the agonizing pain and helplessness you are experiencing for that long unless we hospitalize you and administer high doses of morphine. Let's try to work your surgery into my schedule before I leave."

"What? That's within two weeks!" I was horrified and shocked. I hobbled out of the examination room like a zombie, and limped toward the receptionist's desk. Even though I had been told by my referring physician that orthopedic surgeons needed to be booked months in advance, this caring surgeon was willing to squeeze me in before his vacation. "Someone must be watching over you or your timing must be incredible," the receptionist cheerfully offered. "Just this morning, a patient postponed his surgery because of a respiratory infection. You could have that surgery appointment in two days."

"Two days?" Even though my back was in agonizing pain, I wasn't emotionally ready for this. I went to the doctor that morning for a consultation and I left with an appointment for surgery! It was surreal.

But sometimes, there is a bigger plan than we can fathom. Sometimes, what seems like a horrible answer to a dilemma can become the best solution to our difficulties. "Trust in the Lord with all your heart and lean not into your own understanding, in all your ways acknowledge him and he will make your paths straight." And now, because of my personal experience I can disclose—"and he can make your back straight, too."

It has been almost ten years since that emotionally draining day. Even though the doctor remarked that it was one of the worst cases of a herniated disk that he had seen in his 25 years of surgery, my back has been pain-free ever since. I owe it to more than being in the capable hands of my skilled Irish surgeon. I walk with a spring in my step and an assurance that someone was indeed watching over me.

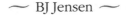 BJ Jensen ~

Oh, My Aching Back!

You Don't Have to Go to War to Have Back Pain

Sergeant Geist's story is reminiscent of many stories I've heard from soldiers who I've treated for back pain. It's physically arduous, sometimes disabling and yes, even potentially deadly, to be a soldier who is stationed far from home. But, you don't have to go to war to have back pain. Many people who have sedentary jobs and have never carried a rifle, never even seen "body armor" much less worn it, and never run from an enemy carrying 60 to 100 pounds of gear, will nevertheless develop severe, perhaps "crippling," back pain.

In fact, the vast majority of us will suffer from back pain at some point in our lives. People are the most likely to suffer between the ages of 20 and 40. However, even though you may be at the greatest risk when you are young and active, getting older doesn't protect you. Aging disks (the "cushions" between the bony vertebrae), arthritis and other problems in the spine may remind you of the passing years. Perhaps not surprisingly, the older you are the more severe and longer lasting the pain may be.

What Does Sex Have to Do With It?

Studies show that back pain doesn't seem to discriminate between the sexes and affects men and women fairly equally. But there do seem to be some sex-related differences. An example where women may be at higher risk for back problems is osteoporosis. While it's true that men get osteoporosis, too, women are particularly susceptible to loss of bone density and strength that can lead to vertebral compression fractures. This may cause them to become shorter and appear somewhat stooped over (commonly known as a dowager's hump).

Men in Western industrialized societies are more apt to have disk problems and this is often treated surgically. Both the problem with their disks and the surgical "solution" may be influenced by the work that they do — with men more likely to be in jobs that require heavy, physical labor and perhaps more interested in pursuing a surgical remedy to get them back to work as quickly as possible.

My Job Is Hurting My Back!

Speaking of jobs and other activities that might predispose someone to back problems, it's probably obvious that jobs that involve lifting, bending, stooping, and so on can take a toll on your back. It's also true that riding in motor vehicles, especially big trucks, construction equipment and even planes that include prolonged sitting combined with vibration, can cause back problems. Lest you think that you are safe in a nice, cushy office, beware — sedentary jobs at the computer are also stressful for backs. Which is why I often counsel young adults who are planning their careers to consider not only their intellectual interests but also how they will physically feel doing their chosen profession year after year. The best kind of a job for your back is one where you don't have to lift too much or sit too much. Backs like to move around but not be too stressed out.

Your neck is the upper part of your back, and it can get stiff simply from daily activities such as sitting at a computer or talking on the phone. Sometimes the stiffness is associated with pain. Your neck is the most flexible portion of your spine. If you have full range of motion, you should be able to:

Forward Flexion: Touch your chin to your chest (or nearly touch it to your chest)

Lateral Flexion: Tilt your head to the side so that it's about halfway to your shoulder

Extension: Look up at the sky

Rotation: Move your head so that you can clearly see oncoming cars when you are driving

When Pain Strikes:
An Exercise to Relieve Neck Pain

Here is a simple, gentle exercise to do when moderate neck pain first strikes. For severe pain, contact your health care provider immediately.

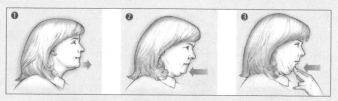

1. Sit in a neutral position, holding your head in a normal resting position.

2. Next, slowly glide your head backward, tucking your chin in until you have pulled your head and chin as far back as they will go. Keep your head level and do not tilt or nod your head. Pull in gently for three to five seconds, then release. Repeat 10 times.

3. For a stronger stretch, gently apply pressure to your chin with your fingers and release. Repeat every two hours as needed.

If this exercise increases your pain, try it lying down on your back. Tuck your chin in and make a double chin. Hold for a second or two and release (your head never leaves the pillow). If pain increases or you develop numbness or tingling, stop and contact your doctor.

Where It Hurts:
Muscles of the Neck

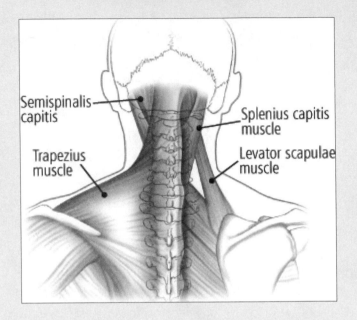

Semispinalis capitis

Splenius capitis muscle

Trapezius muscle

Levator scapulae muscle

The posterior (rear) neck muscles do the lion's share of work in supporting the weight of your head while tilting and turning. Pain can result when an injury strains or tears your neck muscles, but more often, aches and pains result when muscles tense and strain to protect neck joints and nerves that have deteriorated. The brawny trapezius muscle is one of the most common sites of neck pain and strain.

Neck Stretching

Perform these exercises gently to the point where you feel a slight stretch but no pain.

Rotation range-of-motion

Start by facing forward. Turn your head slowly to one side. Hold three seconds and return to the original position. Turn your head slowly to the other side. Hold three seconds and return to the original position. Repeat 10 times.

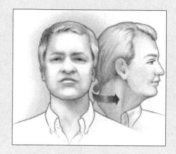

Side bending range-of-motion

Face forward and let your head bend slowly to the side. Hold three seconds and repeat to the other side. Repeat 10 times. Do this exercise slowly and gently.

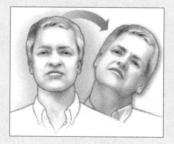

Neck Strengthening

Front neck muscles:

This exercise can be done in a sitting position—at the office, for example—or lying down with your knees bent and feet flat on the floor. Place your palm on your forehead and press gently as you try to bring your chin to your chest; your neck muscles will tighten without your head moving. Hold for a count of three to five seconds. Repeat 10 times.

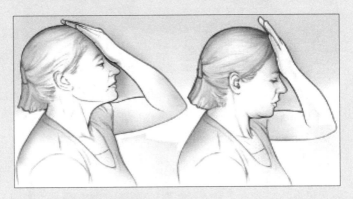

Rear neck muscles:

Place one or both hands behind your head and use them to resist as you press your head backward. Hold for a count of three to five. Repeat 10 times.

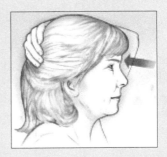

Neck Strengthening

Side neck muscles:

Place your right palm on the right side of your head, using it to resist as you try to bend your right ear toward your shoulder. Hold for a count of 10. Repeat on the left.

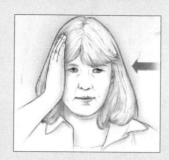

Rotation muscles (not shown):

Place your right hand on the right side of your head. Try to rotate your head to the right, resisting with your hand. Hold for a count of three to five. Repeat on the left. Repeat 10 times.

Shoulder Strengthening

Shoulder blade retractions

Stand up straight with your arms at your sides. Squeeze your shoulder blades together for a count of four and release. Repeat 10 times.

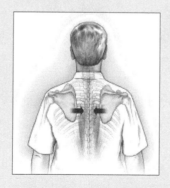

Shoulder Strengthening (continued)

Shoulder strengthener

Secure an elastic exercise band (available at sports and fitness stores) to a sturdy post or railing at waist level. With arms extended, hold the ends of the elastic taut. Pull back slowly, bending your elbows at waist level and squeezing your shoulder blades together. 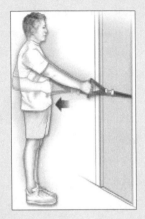 Return slowly to the starting position. Perform three sets of 10 repetitions. Rest one minute between sets.

All figures in Chapter 1 are reprinted with permission from the Harvard Health Publications Special Health Report: Neck and Shoulder Pain (2009)

As people age, they often lose some range of motion. Losing a little is okay, but significant restrictions in neck range of motion can be problematic for daily activities such as driving. On the other hand, sometimes the neck is stretched too far, and this can injure various spinal structures. For example, in a whiplash injury the head is forcibly pushed to the extremes of forward flexion and extension. This causes injury. Too much motion can be harmful, even when it's not associated with trauma. Your neck is only designed to move so far. Pushing it beyond its limits may cause problems.

So, when it comes to neck pain and most other types of pain that involve motion of your body, it's important to stay active and keep things moving well but not overly stretch beyond a normal range of motion. Certainly trauma is one reason why people have neck and back injuries, but sitting for hours on the computer is the cause of many visits to doctors' offices.

Maybe I Can Blame My Parents for My Pain

Some of my patients tell me that they knew they were going to have back problems, because it "runs in my family." Just how much does heredity play a role in back pain? Well, that's a good question and one that is not always simple to answer. Some people may have a genetic susceptibility or "weakness" in certain spinal structures that may predispose them to having back problems. There also is a hereditary link in some back conditions such as ankylosing spondylitis (an inflammatory arthritis that affects men more than women and tends to run in families).

Your family and the environment that you grew up in may also influence your back. For instance, if you grew up in a family that had big meals and relaxed by watching TV after dinner versus a family that ate light meals and went for a hike before dark, these habits—either good or not so good—may influence you now and therefore affect your back.

While there are some genetic and environmental factors that may play a role in back pain, I think it's good to remember that just because someone in your family has back problems doesn't mean that you have the same (or even a very similar) back. This means that there may be treatments that work for you that someone in your family may have unsuccessfully tried. Your back is your own. And this book is both an inspirational guide as well as a back owner's manual!

The Myth of Perfect Posture

Having perfect posture won't keep you from experiencing stiffness and even pain, because your body wants to move. However, many people spend time on the computer, phone and reading at home and work. While improving your posture won't take the place of moving around, it does help when you need to use your arms for a period of time to type or hold a phone or book. Here are some things you can try to better support your upper body. (Hint: even if you don't have neck pain, these are great tips to put your body in a better position and avoid future injury):

1. Support your arms. This is especially important if you use the computer. It's very stressful on your body to have your arms held out in front of you for any period of time. The muscles in your upper and mid back have to contract for long periods of time to hold that position.

    Try this: hold your arms in front of you as if you were typing on the computer. Feel how the muscles in your back are working when you hold your arms in the typing position. Now put your arms in your lap and relax those muscles. Try this a few times until you can really feel the muscles working. Spending 20 minutes at the computer means that those muscles must contract for that period of time. If you are at the computer longer, your muscles work harder. Many people don't have the upper body strength to tolerate this kind of stress on their muscles, so they develop neck and mid back pain.

There are really two solutions to the problem of too much stress on your muscles. The first is to increase strength by doing specific exercises. The second is to decrease the stress on your muscles. When it comes to decreasing stress, there are two options—do less or support more. You can decide whether doing less is an option. Either way, consider offering your upper body more support. One way to do this on the computer is to place a pillow on your lap so that your forearms are supported. Avoid direct pressure over your elbow (where the ulnar nerve is most superficial—you have probably felt the ulnar nerve tingle when you hit your "funny bone" in the past). More sophisticated solutions include ergonomically designed forearm rests (also sometimes called data arms).

2. Use a speakerphone or telephone earset. Even if you don't hold the phone between your neck and shoulder so that your hands are free, it's stressful on your neck to hold the phone up to your ear. Try it without your phone. Pretend you are holding your phone and bring your hand up to your ear. Now, hold that position for the length of a short phone call (say 5-10 minutes). How comfortable does that really feel when you have to hold your arm in that position (and also engage many of the muscles that support your arm, shoulder and neck/back)? Most people don't realize how sustained muscle contractions promote neck pain when they are talking on the phone, but they do. So, go hands-free by using a speakerphone or an earset.

3. Avoid bifocals. You don't really have to throw away your prescription glasses, but if you do wear bifocals think about how you are positioning your neck in order to see. Are you moving your neck into awkward positions so that you are able to see things better? If so, that's probably not helping a sore neck.

4. Use a bookstand. If you love to read, you probably never noticed that it puts stress on your neck muscles to hold a book or an e-reader. This is another thing to try without the actual object. Hold our arms in front of you as if you were reading. Now, keep your arm(s) there for 5-10 minutes. Is that comfortable? Probably not. If you like to read, then it's likely you are holding this position for a lot longer than 5-10 minutes—the whole time engaging your arm, shoulder and neck/back muscles. Instead, try using a bookstand or a pillow on the tabletop or your lap to let your muscles relax.

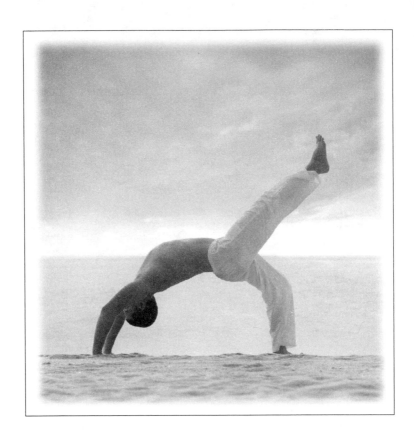

Chapter 2
This Really Hurts!

Uh Oh

Bounce! Bounce! Bounce! It was the summer of 1968. I was bouncing on the large trampolines at the Asbury Park boardwalk. The sea air was blowing in from the Atlantic Ocean just a few hundred yards away and the smell of popcorn and cotton candy permeated the air. Ahhhh... summer time! The world was perfect on this first day of summer vacation! That is until I was flat on my back with a terrible wrench, the worst pain I had experienced in my ten years.

Back at the rental cottage Mom gave me a couple of aspirin to ease the pain and I drifted off into slumber. The next morning I was told there was no lazing around in bed even if I was sore, so I slowly, painfully donned my new bathing suit and moved very deliberately as we made our way to the beach. Once there I planted my feet in the sand where the waves were crashing at mid-chest level in order to feel the rhythmic push and pull which seemed to loosen the pinched nerves and muscles. Once tired of standing in the water I lay down on the hot sand, which soothed the aches.

Before our vacation was complete ten days later I was back to running and playing with the other kids. I could now look back on that evening at the trampolines thinking how silly I must have looked flailing around like a fish out of water while trying to make my legs work and crying through tears of pain.

What a humiliating memory, but little did I know there was more in store.

Fast forward to my rambunctious and rebellious late teenage years in Provo, Utah. One, two, twist, bend down, then up, untwist and repeat on the other side. I was doing windmill toe touches as part of my morning exercise routine when I sneezed and ended up on the floor unable to move, home alone and with a phone clear across the room. My legs wouldn't move and I was once again helpless as shooting stars were blazing in front of my eyes from the pain. The memory of the trampoline came flooding back to me! It took six weeks for me to get back to normal after that incident.

Once again jump forward. I was the single parent of a three-year-old, living in New York City. It was a cold, wet March day as we made our way home on the A train to upper Manhattan from midtown. The train was full and there were no seats so I grasped my son's little hand firmly while hanging on to the overhead strap with the other hand. We were rhythmically swaying with the movement of the train when once again—ouch! I would have fallen right then but there was nowhere to fall since there were bodies pressed tightly all around me.

As the train car emptied a little more at each stop I found myself sinking to my knees. No one offered assistance or even asked if there was anything wrong. When we got to our station I crawled out of the train car onto the platform, desperately clutching my son's hand. He didn't understand what had happened and thought we were playing a game so he crawled along next to me. Thank God for the innocence of children.

The platform and the long tunnel we had to exit from the 191st Street station were wet, muddy and filthy. Leaving the tunnel we still had three blocks to go before reaching our apartment. The rain was now a downpour, so the sidewalks and streets we had to cross were even wetter, muddier and filthier than the tunnel. Luckily my son was adventurous and the tears streaming down my face from the pain were mingling with the rain so he didn't realize our predicament. My stockings were torn to shreds, our hands and knees were filthy, our clothes were drenched from the rain and tears were still streaming down my face. A kindly neighbor held the main door for us and then held the elevator and assisted us to our apartment on the third floor. She unlocked the door for us and then helped me to undress and get into the tub. She fed my son, put him to bed and even brought me a plate of food. I soaked in the tub until the pain subsided enough that I could stand up and go to bed. It took me a few months to recover from that one.

Two years later I was riding in an elevator when the power went out and the elevator abruptly jolted to a stop. Again, it took a few months to recover.

Over the years I have had continued episodes of intense pain and debilitating muscle spasms. I've learned that I will eventually recover from each flare-up. I live a full life these days in a small, rural Idaho town. I enjoy hunting, fishing, hiking, horseback riding and gardening, but I am always aware of anything that sets off a twitch or pain in my lower back. I offer daily prayers of gratitude to the doctors and therapists who have helped me relieve my pain over the years and also those who have taught me techniques such as visualization, meditation and guided imagery to assist me in my desire to refrain from using prescription painkillers. My back problems are something that I have learned to accept and manage, and I go on with a full life despite them.

— Laura D. Hollingshead —

As Strong as an Oak Tree

"How is your back?" seems to be the way most people greet me now. They don't say, "Hi, good to see you! What have you been going?" Nope, they ask, "How is your back?"

I'd been galloping my horse over the crest of a hill and there was a sudden sharp drop into a deep ravine. The horse stopped but I didn't. I was thrown over the horse's head and down into the ravine. I hit the ground hard. My back felt as if it was on fire and I could barely move my left leg without screaming. I was miles from anyone, with no cell phone, and no one knew where I was. I live alone so it could have been a week or more before anyone noticed I was missing. I had no choice but to crawl out of the ravine, pull myself back up into the saddle and ride my horse home. It was a long and extremely painful ride.

It was six hours after the injury before I could get medical help. I was in agony. The doctor said nothing was broken, my spine was slightly crooked, and one vertebra was knocked out of alignment, but he didn't think anything could or should be done about it. I was to let my body heal naturally. He said to use crutches until my leg stopped hurting.

I hobbled around on crutches for three weeks, then hobbled around without them for another three weeks. I slowly regained the use of my leg and didn't waddle like a duck anymore. I could finally put my left foot flat on the floor. I'd been tiptoeing on it since the fall.

My back still felt like it was on fire, especially if I bent over to pick up something. I also had a knot the size of a golf ball in the middle of my back and if I sat in a hard-backed chair or bumped the lump, it would send a sharp pain through my back.

My friends suggested a back brace, a variety of treatments and medications, and a different doctor. They warned me that a "woman my age" needed to be careful because if I fell again I could be crippled or paralyzed. After all, I was sixty-eight years old and not a kid anymore. I couldn't just go around doing the things I did when I was young.

I became careful and fearful. I took smaller steps when I walked. I sat in soft chairs. My back became an excuse not to do things. What if I fell? What if I got hurt again? What if that crooked vertebra decided to slip out of place? What if?

Friends still greeted me with, "How's your back?" I felt like there was more to me than just my back and began feeling like my back had a social life of its own. It could start going to parties by itself while the rest of me stayed home. I was no longer a woman—I was a woman with a back problem. Or maybe I was a back problem with a woman attached.

When people asked me how I was doing, I'd tell them "I'm doing okay I guess. I'm 90% healed," or "I'm 99% healed." I wondered if someone asked me if I was alive I would answer, "I'm 90% alive" or "I'm 99% alive." It was as if I had to maintain a bit of my injury to keep my membership in the club that I seemed to have joined.

I was sympathetic to those who were suffering from various injuries and ailments but it seemed every contact with my friends turned into an "organ recital" where we all complained about what was wrong with our organs. All we seemed to talk about was a grocery list of illnesses, medications and doctors.

My back pain had become a "pain in the neck." I wasn't enjoying life. I decided to do something about it.

As soon as I woke up every morning I told myself how great I felt. I stopped "being careful." I took longer strides when I walked. I stood up straighter. My back was healing but I had allowed well-meaning people to make me think of myself as "the woman with the back problem." I decided I would no longer discuss my health or my back with anyone.

I began to picture my spine as the trunk of a tree, my head, arms and legs were the branches. I pictured a strong, sturdy oak tree, capable of supporting its limbs and withstanding any storm. Instead of thinking my back was weak because it had been injured in a fall, I began to think how amazingly strong it had been to endure such a bad fall and not break.

I began to believe I had an incredibly strong spine. After all, it had survived a trauma. It was still a little crooked but it functioned normally. The lump on my back was getting smaller and would disappear in another month.

I found my courage again and began doing everything I loved. I started riding my horse again; I went ice skating and hiking. The less my back hurt, the less I thought about it, or perhaps it worked the other way around and the less I thought about my back the less it hurt.

Will I gallop my horse across the hills again? Yes, because I love riding. Will I fall off my horse again? Well, I hope not, but I might. Will I fall down if I go ice-skating? Probably, because I'm not very good at ice-skating, but I enjoy it. Will I live my life in constant fear of what "might" happen? No, definitely not. I will live my life to the fullest every day. I will not be foolish, but I will not be "careful" or "fearful" and I will not live half of a life. Life is a great adventure, or it is nothing.

If anyone asks me how I'm doing, I'll say, "I'm doing great!"

— April Knight —

Carry My Brother

As an eighteen-year-old college student, being frugal was vital, so I had rushed over to the flashing blue light that indicated purses were drastically reduced. I didn't quite make it to the blue light, although I could see it from where I lay flat out on the cold floor as other shoppers walked over me. My back had given out one more time. I was in good shape, young, and healthy otherwise, but my back had carried more than its share of weight in my young life and it was beginning to fail me.

My younger brother Scott could not walk or talk due to his cerebral palsy. I loved Scott dearly and carried him wherever I could, including playgrounds, mountaintops, and church. This was back in the 1960's, way before public places had to be handicapped-accessible. My back was my brother's carriage and I gladly showed him all that I could. He was my brother, my best friend and I would carry him joyfully for as long as our childhood allowed.

And now, lying there in pain, I thought of my brother. How he would laugh at me now, looking up at others who hurried past me. The store manager came and asked what I was doing. I explained to him I was having a back spasm and I just needed to rest a bit. He was sympathetic, but he told me I could only lie there ten minutes.

I did then what I continue to do today, forty years later, to help myself cope with back pain—I used imagery. I closed my eyes and calmly envisioned happy places, places of comfort and peace, such as a rolling stream, a beautiful ocean scene, soft flower petals falling on me, and the faces of people I loved. Mentally moving myself from a painful place to a peaceful one decreases my back pain and gives me some control over my body. It does not relieve the pain entirely, but it helps me to feel a sense of connection between my body and my mind, a place where hopeful thoughts take root.

The ten minutes passed and my imagery time was up. I felt well enough to walk again. I slowly got up and smiled. There were still purses on that table and the blue light was still flashing. I made sure to purchase a small purse, one that could hold my bare necessities. After all, a large, heavy purse can harm one's back. And besides, I already had something big to carry: my brother's love.

— Malinda Dunlap Fillingim —

I Can't Move
My Head!

I carry a heavy backpack to and from school each day and I dance for four hours a week, so my neck gets sore sometimes. Very sore. My neck has always been sensitive, and it doesn't help that I am a petite girl, a bit smaller than my classmates. Usually, my mom, who is a doctor and the author of this book, helps my neck feel better by giving me a quick massage.

One morning, in third grade, I woke up and my neck felt different—worse than ever. The night before, my neck had been a little bit sore. But that morning, I couldn't even move it; it was tilted to the side and stuck in that position. It hurt a lot. Every time I tried to move it, I felt a sharp pain. When I told my mom, who is a physiatrist, she explained that I had torticollis, a condition in which the head is turned to one side and cannot be moved to the other side, along with muscle spasms.

Hearing that I had torticollis made me nervous. Was I going to have this condition for life?

My mother helped my neck by stretching it, that is to say pulling it gently so that it would straighten out. I had to resist the urge to squeal in pain when she did that. I also had a special kind of massage where I lay down and my mom put her hands behind my head and the back of my neck and tenderly massaged it. When I went to school, I had a lot of trouble talking to the other kids and the teacher, because I could only face in one direction. But with my mom helping me stretch my neck out, after about three days, it felt entirely better.

I was so relieved when I could finally move my neck normally again. I now take it for granted that I can move my neck without difficulty, but I will never forget the time I had torticollis.

~ Anna Rose Silver, age 11 ~

This Really Hurts!

I can vividly imagine Laura bouncing on a trampoline, hair blowing in the wind, ocean waves rhythmically keeping time with her youthful energy. Beachgoers are milling all around, scratchy sand between their toes, snow cones dripping, and the sun gently warming their smiling faces.

How does this fun summertime adventure, that most of us can imagine as we recall our own childhood beach memories, suddenly turn into a horrifying event in which "I am flat on my back with a terrible wrench, the worst pain I had experienced in my 10 years?" Laura's story highlights several important points:

1. Back pain can start at any point during your life.
2. Once you have back pain, it's likely that there will be flare-ups at different times.
3. Sometimes you can point to a specific injury or way that you move that caused the pain to start (and this can give you clues about how to avoid back pain in the future).

In Laura's case, her first episode of back pain was when she was around 10 years old. The pain started during forceful movements that included bouncing as well as twisting and turning. The second time she had an episode of pain, it occurred when she was performing bending and twisting motions while doing exercises. The third time this happened she was on a train and her body was again in motion — swaying. Although, Laura can point to specific events that caused her pain, there were undoubtedly many times in between these episodes in which she performed bending, twisting and other motions and these didn't cause pain. It's difficult to say exactly what happened that caused these painful episodes, but it was probably a combination of things that occurred simultaneously — like a "perfect storm."

Your Back Anatomy

The back is a pretty complicated and confusing part of your anatomy. One of the reasons it can be very hard for doctors to pinpoint the precise part of the spine that is causing someone pain is that there are quite a few structures that may be problematic. But, it's easier to break it down into six parts and to consider each part when trying to diagnose the cause of someone's back pain.

1. Bones
2. Disks
3. Joints
4. Ligaments
5. Muscles
6. Nerves

The first part of your back is the long line of bones (vertebrae) stacked on top of each other. Each vertebra has a cylindrical shaped body with a bony ring attached to its back. If you put your hand on your spine, you can feel the spinous process of each vertebra. The lumbar vertebrae are in the low back, and they carry most of your body weight and are subjected to the greatest stress when you twist, turn, bend, stand, walk, run and

A Closer Look at Your Lumbar Vertebrae

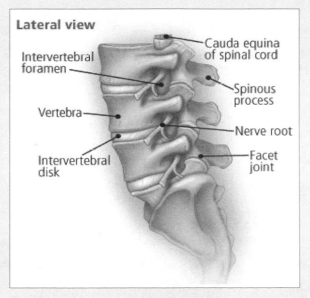

Lateral view

Cauda equina of spinal cord

Intervertebral foramen

Spinous process

Vertebra

Nerve root

Intervertebral disk

Facet joint

Each vertebra has a cylindrical body with a bony ring attached to its back surface as well as bony processes that project out in different directions from this ring. Intervertebral disks, tucked between each pair of vertebrae, serve as shock absorbers.

A Closer Look at Your Lumbar Vertebrae (continued)

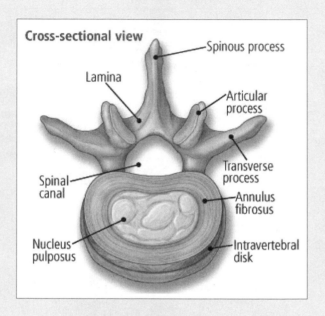

Cross-sectional view

Spinous process

Lamina

Articular process

Transverse process

Spinal canal

Annulus fibrosus

Nucleus pulposus

Intravertebral disk

Each intervertebral disk has a gelatinous central part, called the nucleus pulposus, and a fibrous covering, called the annulus fibrosus. Each vertebra normally has seven processes (five are shown above; the other two are obscured in this illustration) that help stabilize your spine.

Reprinted with permission from the Harvard Health Publications Special Health Report: Low Back Pain (2010) lift objects. There are five lumbar vertebrae, and not surprisingly, they are the biggest and strongest of the bones in your back.

In between the vertebrae are disks. Your disks are spongy and have the same shape as the cylindrical body of the vertebrae (which makes sense, because this means that the disk fits nicely in between the two vertebral bones). Sometimes the disks pop out a bit—sort of like an inflated balloon can change shape when you apply pressure to one end. There are lots of terms to describe discs that become misshapen, and even doctors don't really agree on which terms to use in every situation. However, when you hear someone say that they have a "bulging disk" or "herniated disk" or "slipped disk" or "ruptured disk" (or something similar), what they are describing is a disk that is misshapen and no longer in the nice cylindrical shape of the vertebrae above and below it. Radiologists often call these disk protrusions or extrusions.

The vertebrae are linked together by ligaments to form joints that allow you to flex, twist and bend to some degree (the joints allow some movement but also restrict movement—if you had too much movement in your spine you'd become very unstable).

The ligaments support your spinal column and allow your back to move, but they don't cause the movement. What causes movement are your muscles. Muscles shorten (contract) and lengthen (expand) to make your back move.

The final category of "back parts" I want to talk about are your nerves. You can think of your nerves as the electrical cord to your muscles—they supply the power to make the muscles work. If the nerves are injured, your muscles get weak and don't work well (as if you pulled the plug on the electrical cord). Probably the most concise way to understand the nerves in the back is to recognize that there is a long column of them that are bundled together like a cord—hence the name spinal cord—that goes from the top to the bottom of your spine.

At the end of the spinal cord the nerves become unbundled but still hang together (like the hair on a horse's tail). These loose nerves at the end of the spinal column are called the *cauda equina*, which means "horse's tail." Along the way, at every level, there are two nerves that branch off called "nerve roots" (one on the right and one on the left). These are the ones that often get pinched when a disk bulges. So, there is the spinal cord that ends in the cauda equina and the nerve roots. Injury to the spinal cord, cauda equina or nerve roots are the most serious problems that doctors worry about.

How to Think Like a Doctor

Taking the example of Laura, it's impossible to go back in time and diagnose the specific structures in the spine that were injured the first time Laura experienced back pain. However, from her reported history in the story, it's likely that it was either her muscles or ligaments or both. The reason I say this is that I'm thinking about each of the six categories and ruling some of them out. Here's what I'm thinking: It's unlikely that Laura broke any bones by jumping on a trampoline (it is possible, but unless she fell off, it's unlikely). Moreover, she healed pretty quickly (by her account in just a few days), and broken bones don't heal that fast. So, it wasn't bone trauma.

Next on my list are disks and nerves. That's a possibility, but disk problems are more common among middle aged and older people. This is because as we age our disks tend to dry out and their shock absorption capabilities become less effective. When disks bulge, they often touch or push a nerve. This causes nerve symptoms such as numbness, tingling and sharp or "electrical" pain down one leg. Again, Laura didn't have these symptoms, so I suspect that her problem didn't involve a disk pressing on a nerve (technically called *radiculopathy*).

Joint pain is usually due to aging. This is a form of arthritis, and the most common cause in the back is *facet arthropathy*. It is possible to develop other joint problems, but an injury to a joint is less likely than muscle strains and ligament sprains — what is often called a "soft tissue injury." Muscle strains and ligament sprains often occur together and may be referred to as a "sprain-strain injury." These soft tissue injuries are not easily seen on imaging studies such as X-rays that mostly demonstrate bone structure and help to rule out fractures. More likely than not, Laura's first injury was a lumbar sprain-strain injury, likely involving stretching and minor trauma to some muscles and ligaments in her back. This is the most common type of back pain and can usually be diagnosed by history and physical examination. This type of injury typically resolves fairly quickly — even without treatment. If it doesn't get better within a couple of weeks, then it's a good idea to check in with a doctor.

In this chapter, I focused on "how to think like a doctor." The critical part of thinking like a doctor is to understand the anatomy and then to know what possible problems there can be in the different parts of the body (or back, in this case). By knowing the anatomy of the back, doctors can listen to a patient's story, examine the patient, and then decide what is the most likely diagnosis. However, there are times when it's not so easy or when the problem is potentially very serious. In the next chapter, I'll discuss when to be worried (or not).

Why Does My Back Hurt?

The actual cause of back pain can vary, as there are many structures in this region of the body that may cause symptoms. In fact, there are so many structures, that are so complex, it's not uncommon that the precise cause of the pain cannot be accurately diagnosed—even with the latest technology and imaging studies. However, if you have neck or low back pain, some of the possible causes include:

- Radiculopathy (due to pressure on a nerve coming from the spine—often caused by a bulging or herniated disk—in the low back this is often called "sciatica")

- Spinal stenosis (this is a narrowing of the bony spinal canal which causes the nerves to be "squeezed")

- Facet arthropathy (this is usually due to aging or "arthritis" of the joints in the spine)

- Sprain/strain (a common cause of low back pain that may be due to injury to multiple structures such as muscles and tendons)

- Tumors (not a common cause of back pain but a worrisome one — a "red flag" for this is pain that awakens you at night)

- Bony fractures (these may be due to trauma or sometimes occur without any injury in people with osteoporosis — a specific type of fracture that sometimes occurs in teen athletes as well as other people is called spondylolysis or spondylolisthesis)

- Infection (this is pretty rare but can be serious — people at risk for infection include those with liver failure, diabetes or AIDS)

- Spinal cord compression (this is also unusual but very worrisome and may be associated with weakness, loss of bowel/bladder control and, in men, problems with erections — cauda equina syndrome occurs below the level of the spinal cord where the nerves bundle together in the spine and can cause similar symptoms)

My Neck Thing

When my daughter wrote about having torticollis for this book, she labeled her word document "Neck Thing." Which is a relatively apt, though not very technical, term for torticollis.

Torticollis has also been called "wryneck" and typically involves the neck twisting with the head tipping to one side while the chin is pointed to the other side. Sometimes this is present at birth (congenital torticollis) and in other people it is acquired later in life. If there is no known reason for it to occur, it is called idiopathic torticollis. Torticollis may be due to a variety of factors including injury to the nervous system or muscles. Spasmodic torticollis is usually classified as a movement disorder and can be quite painful and debilitating.

It is usually easier to treat torticollis in children and before it becomes chronic. Treatment options vary, depending on the cause and duration of symptoms. Usually the treatment includes gentle stretching, heat and massage. Sometimes oral or injected medications are used. For more severe or chronic cases, botulinum toxin injections may be helpful. Rarely surgery is indicated.

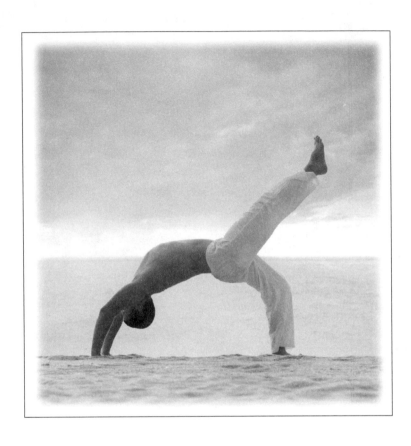

Chapter 3
I'm Afraid This Is Serious

A Healthier Lifestyle with Spondilitis

I t may be a strange way to put it, but my back had always been my "Achilles' heel." As a child I remember being plagued by an aching back and aching limbs. "Growing pains," said the local physician, with a dismissive wave of his hands, as I wept my way through the excruciating pain that racked my bones throughout childhood. This was in the early Sixties, when painkillers in India were not considered safe for children, especially for long-term use.

Could it be attributed to genetics? My brother, two years my senior, also suffered from backaches so severe that even during his school days he was advised to sit on a specially constructed hard wooden chair, and had to wear a back brace. My memories of my maternal grandmother are wrapped around a soft-spoken lady who otherwise beautiful, was bent double at the waist. My mother suffered the same affliction, and even before she had reached sixty, was bent like a leaning-forward L. I often wondered if I would suffer the same way.

While the backaches retreated in my late teens, they were back with renewed vigor when I had my baby at twenty-three. As I sat up for successive nights, rocking, feeding and soothing a bawling infant, my back took a severe beating. I developed a chronic low back pain, which continued even when my daughter reached her teens. Even with regular walks, advised by doctors, the pain never really went away. A low back pain was my constant companion. It became worse when we were posted to regions that had high atmospheric levels of humidity, but with a husband in the Air Force, this was an occupational hazard we had to accept.

A decade and a half later, I began to experience additional symptoms. My shoulders became achy and sore, and it became increasingly difficult and painful to turn my neck or lift my arms. Soon, I began to experience shooting pains radiating from my neck, right up to my eyes. Matters came to a head one evening, when I could not raise my arms even to take off my dress.

"Acute cervical spondylitis!" pronounced the orthopedic surgeon the next day. I had a choice between an unwieldy neck brace or an hour of traction, followed by deep heat therapy and massage at the physio-therapy department, every day. I would have to follow up at home with a regimen of special exercises thrice a day. When I mentioned my low back pain, the doctor diagnosed it as lumbar spondilitis and added a few more exercises to my routine.

This was precious time that I had to squeeze in between my teaching job, housework and a little craft-production that I did from home, but I kept it up. A month later, the physio-therapist pronounced that since I'd been an earnest student, I could stop the visits to the physio-therapy department. "But the exercises must continue. You have to do them every day for the rest of your life, or you may even need surgery," he warned me, explaining that exercise would help strengthen the muscles and joints.

I was lucky to get a wonderful physio-therapist, who took the time to explain the nature and treatment of the ailment. He advised me to throw away my fluffy pillow. "It's best to sleep without one, but if that is uncomfortable, use a flat one, not thicker than a plump pizza," was his advice. The soft mattress had to be replaced with a firm one. I was told to give up my stitching, knitting and other crafting hobbies since they involved bending my head forward, a posture that pressed on crucial spinal nerves.

Today, twenty-one years later, I follow the entire gamut of exercises for six days of the week. I start with simple calisthenics to warm up, followed by isometric exercises and neck rotations for the cervical spondilitis. Next come some stretches, bends and yoga poses (Boat Pose, Cat-Cow Pose and Plough Pose) to help the lumbar spondilitis. After a hysterectomy, on the advice of a gynecologist, I even added a few rounds of Kegels to strengthen the pelvic muscles. Forty minutes of this routine every morning helps to tone up the muscles of the upper body.

In the evening, the lower muscles get their share of exercise with a brisk four-kilometer walk. Menopause brings with it an additional risk of osteoporosis, which could result in weakening and bending of the spine. Sunshine was necessary to keep this at bay, so I factored that in by walking in bright sunshine and doing a bit of gardening, too.

Since my life would be barren without my knitting, crochet

and embroidery, I devised a method to help me continue. I use a small pillow on my knees to raise the height of the material I'm working on, and for additional support, I use two small pillows under each elbow.

While backaches may certainly have a physiological reason, medical experts are increasingly linking emotional and mental stress to tightening of muscles and nerves, which could result in backaches. While some healers advise meditation, I found my own ways to de-stress. I took up volunteer work—my husband and I make music. We visit cancer patients, disabled people, senior citizens, orphanages. Singing, laughing and talking to them, being able to bring a spark to their eyes and a smile to their lips, gives me a warm oozy feeling, and loosens up the knots in my joints. It's like a restful gentle massage.

And my most important de-stressor—talking to my Creator. Every morning as I get up, I thank the Almighty for the new day and new opportunity; and every night along with the day's review, I give thanks for the many happy hours which were gifted to me that day. It doesn't take more than five minutes, but it creates a soft restful glow. As I move towards my sixtieth birthday, I begin to think that the spondilitis has given me a richer and healthier lifestyle—physically, emotionally and spiritually.

Does the cervical or lumbar spondilitis still bother me? In these two decades, I've had only a single relapse. This was five years ago, when I went to visit my daughter. When my neck, shoulder and arms became severely achy, I visited the hospital right next door, and the resident physio-therapist confirmed that it was my old friend (spondilitis) visiting me again. While a week of the usual routine of traction, heat and massage took care of the matter, I was at a loss why it had recurred. It didn't take long to spot the culprit. Forgetting previous advice, I was using a beautiful plump pillow again! The moment I got rid of it, my pain too vanished. And now I take care never to repeat that mistake.

— Mita Banerjee —

Plenty

My last day of teaching with the school district was on a Friday. The family came to celebrate with me on Sunday, and by 8:00 p.m. an ambulance was rushing me to the emergency room. By 10:00 I was being slowly moved into the dark cave of medical machinery for an MRI to determine what was causing the shattering pain in my back and right leg.

I tried to suppress my panic and fear, but I was anxiously grieving for all the plans I had for that summer. No hiking. No teaching a summer class at the university. No trips. No beginning of the new phase of life that had been beckoning me to go do something for the Lord. I tried to put on a brave smile for the technician.

I closed my eyes as I was rolled into the narrow world of the MRI machine. I heard the technician remind me to try not to move. I prayed between gulps of breath. Then, gradually, with my eyes closed I became unaware of the tightness of the enclosure, the possibility of claustrophobia, or the caution to be extremely still. Instead, under my eyelids I saw light. I felt bathed in it, warmed by it and comforted. I knew with a deep knowing that there was a kind of healing already taking place. Even in great pain, something was healing. When I was informed later that I needed a second MRI that night, I found myself almost smiling in anticipation of this sweet and totally unexpected gift of consolation and love. Again, there was the light, and warmth and sweetness of knowing that something beautiful was happening even though I was hurting.

Later, the weary doctor informed me that I had a ruptured disc, nerve damage and a small tumor on my spine. Several days later he performed surgery and pronounced it successful.

I returned on unwieldy crutches to my small three-level townhome to find that my daughters had moved a mattress into the middle of the living room floor near the TV. It was surrounded by items I would need: some books, a telephone, Kleenex, and pain pills. With no way to manage stairs, I wouldn't have access to a bath or shower, my bedroom, my office and computer, or my closet of clothes.

My new world would be anything I could reach from the mattress. My daughters would visit and bring me delicious cold drinks, because the refrigerator might as well have been in another country. In the fog of medications I wondered if I would ever walk again, because even with crutches I could barely stand. Within my small world I would sleep, read, pray and try to keep track of the days.

My right leg continued to be numb, but as the days went by I was able to start hobbling from mattress to couch to refrigerator to the small guest bathroom. I was an adventurer in my own home, rediscovering how wonderful it is to be able to move about at all! There were unexplored paths and familiar ones. As well as the physical distances to re-discover, I took inner journeys and found neglected memories to re-live, stories to be recalled, dear faces to be remembered and blessings to be counted.

Yes, something transformative had happened when I had those two MRIs. I hadn't been promised that I would heal perfectly or that I would be able to do all I had planned to do. I had been given a greater gift: the knowledge that no matter what happened I would not be alone and I would be given what was necessary for that day, for that moment. I would begin to see my world through new eyes. It was enough.

In the fall, as I continued to recover, a friend gave me a small painting. It simply features a bowl of lovely fruit on a checked tablecloth with the word "plenty" painted below it. Every day I look upon that little piece of art and recognize the deep truth of it. My leg didn't heal fully. Especially in the mornings I walk hunched over with little tentative steps. It doesn't matter. When I thought I had lost so much I was given a gift of plenty. Within the confines of the MRI where I could have been consumed with fear, I had been given warmth and consolation. Within my small living room, residing on the island of my mattress, I had traveled within my heart and memories and found riches. I had been given the "plenty" of my daughters' love, devotion and compassion.

By nature I can let shortsighted anxiety fill spaces in my heart that I would prefer to have inhabited by optimism and hope. In beautiful churches I have tried to leave my worries behind, and stop fretting over a future that isn't mine to know. Yet, it was during an MRI, vulnerable and in pain, that I found a different kind of cathedral where I was allowed to see that within even the smallest moment, there is plenty.

~ Caroline S. McKinney ~

Twist
and Shout

I'd never really understood what people meant when they claimed they'd thrown out their backs. I'd thrown out faded towels, broken alarm clocks and even coffee grounds, but never my back... nor any other part of my anatomy. I didn't get it.

And then one day I did. As a Peace Corps Volunteer, I'd been flying back to Belize City from a conference in Trinidad. When the plane taxied to a stop, I jumped up and bent down to retrieve my duffle bag from under my seat. As I straightened up, I shrieked with pain, startling my fellow passengers, and especially the flight attendants, who hustled down the aisle towards my side.

"What's wrong?"

I was crying so hard I could hardly get the words out. "I've done something bad to the right side of my back," I finally managed.

They called for a wheelchair to transport me to the baggage claim. Lucky for me, the Peace Corps driver had already pulled up at the curb, just as we'd prearranged. I couldn't tolerate sitting outdoors for long in the sultry 100-degree tropical heat.

"Going home to Regent Street?" he asked, helping me from the wheelchair to the car.

"No. I have to stop by the office first and see Nurse Jackie."

Nurse Jackie had been the Peace Corps Medical Officer since I'd been a Volunteer. She gave us our gamma globulin shots, dispensed our Aralen prophylactic pills to guard against malaria, and assessed us for the usual array of scrapes, bruises and fevers that seemed to befall us continually.

"What'd you do, girl?" Nurse Jackie frowned as she watched me creep across the floor.

"I hurt my back somehow. I don't understand it. I only reached under the plane seat to get my bag."

"Were you standing up, and then leaned to the side?"

"Yes, of course."

"Done say it," Nurse Jackie commented, as she slipped into Belizean Creole, shaking her head.

I felt relieved immediately, because "done say it" translated into "Okay, I hear you, I've got your number." Nurse Jackie would know what to do. Maybe I'd be able to stand up straight once again, or sit down, or even take a few unaided steps.

"I'm giving you a muscle relaxant and I'll ask the driver to take you home. Get in bed and stay there as much as you can for the next couple of days. You've pulled a muscle in your lower back and I'll tell you exactly how you did it."

"I just leaned over to the side," I sputtered.

"That's not all. You didn't make your nose follow your toes. Never twist or bend your body when you're lifting anything. It doesn't matter how heavy it is. You can throw out your back just by reaching down from your chair to pick up a dropped pencil. And if you're standing up, make sure your nose and toes always point in the same direction."

For the next two days I played invalid, dozing atop my sheet, sipping limeade and reading a Jonathan Kellerman paperback. I still suffered whenever I tried to stand up. It continued to take me ten minutes to inch my way down the hall to the bathroom. But by the third day, time, rest and the muscle relaxants finally combined to get me back on my feet.

For the remainder of my Peace Corps service in Belize, no matter what I did, I always made certain my nose followed my toes. I'd remind myself as I washed my laundry in the bathtub and hung it on the line, as I plucked a basket of mangoes from the trees in my yard, as I stooped over to pat a preschooler on the head. Nose follows toes. It became my mantra.

It still is, and I've Nurse Jackie to thank. Done say it! She had my number, and she had my back.

— Terri Elders —

I'm Afraid This Is Serious

The word *pain* comes from the French *peine* and Latin *poena*, which mean "a penalty or punishment." The etymology of "pain" unfortunately reflects the historical belief that suffering was divinely imposed as penance for sinful acts. Many people still adhere to this idea, either willingly or not, and when they become ill ask themselves, "What have I done to deserve this?"

Saint Augustine claimed that the greatest evil is physical pain. Thankfully, over time we have developed many medications and other therapies that help to alleviate this evil. However, it's no secret that despite significant advances in pain medicine, patients continue to suffer much more than they should. This is why relieving pain, and thus unnecessary suffering, has recently become such an important component of good healthcare that *rating pain is now formally called the fifth vital sign* (after temperature, blood pressure and heart and respiratory rates).

As a physiatrist, I spend a lot of time evaluating pain symptoms. Are they serious? What should I do to investigate the symptoms? How should I treat them?

Every time someone comes into my office with back pain, the first thing I do is listen to them explain what happened. Sometimes, they'll tell me a very dramatic story, such as April shared, when she was thrown from her horse. Other times, the story is simply bending or twisting the wrong way. Still other times, my patients really don't know what is causing their pain. In the chart, I will write down, "No inciting event."

The next thing I want to know is more information about the pain itself. Since, I can't see pain on physical examination, I have to rely on the patient to explain what he or she is experiencing. Pain is real, but only the patient is able to describe how it feels. In order to better understand patients' pain experience, doctors are taught to ask a series of specific questions. We learn these in medical school, and they should be part of every initial consultation by a doctor who is treating someone for back pain. The information doctors need to know to make the right diagnosis includes:

- Location—Where is the pain and does it radiate anywhere?
- Quality—What does the pain feel like? Is it burning, sharp, etc.?
- Intensity—On a scale of 0-10 with 10 being intolerable, how bad is it at its best and worst?
- Frequency—When does it occur?
- Duration—How long does it last?
- Aggravating Components—What makes it worse?
- Alleviating Components—What makes it better?

Is My Back Pain an Emergency?

When I'm listening to the patient respond to each question, I'm constantly thinking about whether there are any "red flags."

Doctors use this phrase to mean "reasons to be really worried and do something right away." There are three main reasons why doctors get really worried. The first reason is that we are concerned that there might be a tumor (either cancer or another type of tumor that is benign). The second one is that we suspect that there may be a bone fracture. The third reason is that we are worried about serious nerve injury (either to the spinal cord, *cauda equina* or nerve roots). Doctors think of "red flags" as either medical emergencies or as potentially serious problems that need a prompt investigation followed by appropriate treatment interventions—depending on the diagnosis.

The red flag symptoms that doctors worry the most about include:

- Recent trauma
- Numbness in your groin or anal area
- Weakness in your legs
- Pain at night, especially if you can't sleep well due to pain
- Pain at rest, especially if it's severe
- Fever
- Urinary or bowel incontinence
- History of cancer or immunocompromised state (e.g., organ transplant, HIV, etc.)

When to Call the Doctor

Most neck pain doesn't stem from anything medically serious, making it safe to try self-care strategies before seeking medical help. However, if your neck pain is so severe you can't sit still, or if it is accompanied by any of the following symptoms, contact a medical professional right away.

- Fever, headache, and neck stiffness. This triad of symptoms might indicate bacterial meningitis, an infection of the spinal cord and brain covering that requires prompt treatment with antibiotics.
- Pain traveling down one arm, especially if the arm or hand is weak, numb, or tingling. Your symptoms might indicate that a herniated cervical disk is pressing on a nerve.
- Loss of bowel or bladder control. This might indicate pressure on the spinal cord or spinal nerve roots, needing immediate attention.
- Extreme instability. If you can suddenly flex or extend your neck much farther than usual, it might indicate a fracture or torn ligaments. This usually occurs only after significant impact or injury, and is more likely to be detected by your doctor or on an X-ray than by your own perception.

- Persistent swollen glands in the neck. Infection or tumor can result in swollen glands and neck pain.
- Chest pain or pressure. A heart attack or inflamed heart muscle can cause neck pain along with more classic heart symptoms.

Reprinted with permission from the Harvard Health Publications Special Health Report: Neck and Shoulder Pain (2010)

As I mentioned, the vast majority of back pain can be diagnosed by history and physical examination. Medical tests, such as imaging studies, should be ordered only when there is a concern about a serious problem such as a fracture, the diagnosis is not clear, there is a progression of symptoms (for example, someone is losing strength in one leg), or the study is needed in order to direct treatment (for example, a doctor should always order imaging studies before recommending surgery).

Diagnosing Back Pain with Medical Tests

There are several types of imaging studies that doctors may order to evaluate back pain. These include:

- **X-rays**—These primarily show the bones in your back. They can give clues about other structures, too, but they don't show the "soft tissues" very well. X-rays are very helpful when diagnosing fractures, changes to bones caused by tumors, infection and certain forms of arthritis. X-rays do involve radiation, but the amount from one set is quite small.

- **Computed Tomography (CT) scans** — CT scans are really sophisticated X-rays that take multiple pictures, each from a slightly different angle. They provide more information about the bones and can show subtle fractures, arthritis and narrowing of the spinal canal (called *spinal stenosis*). CT scans do not show the soft tissues, such as muscles, ligaments and nerves, very well. Similar to standard X-rays, CT scans do involve some radiation. So, it's best to order CT scans only when it's really necessary to see the bony structures in more detail than a plain X-ray will show.

- **Magnetic Resonance Imaging (MRI)** — MRIs use electromagnetic waves to create images of your tissues. Not everyone can have an MRI. For example, if you have metal in your body, the magnet from the MRI may damage the tissues around the metal. MRIs show soft tissue structures the best, such as a bulging disk that may be pressing on a nerve. Though this is not always true, you can think of a CT scan as showing the bones better and an MRI as demonstrating the soft tissues better. So, a doctor will usually order one or the other (not usually both) depending on which structures he or she wants to look at most closely.

- **Myelography**—This form of diagnostic imaging involves injecting fluid (a radiographic dye) into the area around the spinal cord and cauda equina and then looking at where it goes with a special X-ray machine called a fluoroscope. Myelography provides information about what the spinal cord, spinal canal, *cauda equina* and other structures look like and whether there is pressure on them for some reason. This imaging study is less commonly used today than it was in the past when CTs and MRIs weren't readily available.

- **Bone scan**—Bone scans are performed by injecting a short-lived radioactive substance into the bloodstream. The bones absorb this substance at different rates—depending on the activity of the cells. A tumor, infection or healing fracture will appear as a "hot spot."

- **Electromyography (EMG) and Nerve Conduction Study (NCS)**—Sometimes both of these tests are referred to as an EMG, but usually an EMG is done together with NCS. The EMG part of the test involves putting thin needles into the muscles and testing them. There are no electrical shocks given during an EMG, usually. The NCS part of the test usually involves surface electrodes that don't pierce the skin. Small electrical shocks are used to see how well the nerves are working. This is an uncomfortable test, so it is usually done when there is a question about the diagnosis — either the cause of the problem or the severity. However, unlike some of the imaging studies, EMGs and NCSs are physiologic tests (so, they don't take pictures, but rather tell the physician what is happening to the muscles and nerves and how well they are working)

In Caroline's case, she likely had an MRI because her doctor was concerned about a serious problem and was considering surgery. This is precisely the kind of situation in which an MRI is recommended. However, just because a doctor orders an imaging test doesn't mean that there will be a serious problem uncovered or that surgery will be necessary. In fact, a lot of times imaging studies are ordered to "rule out" a serious problem and the results don't show anything too concerning.

Each of these structures may play a role in serious and not so serious back pain problems and sometimes more than one is causing pain. However, as the stories in the next chapter demonstrate (and you may already know this from personal experience), all back pain can be debilitating and hard to live with.

Pain Talks to You

What would it be like to live without pain? For many, this would be a huge relief. However, the reality of a pain-free life is very different for those with a condition called "congenital insensitivity to pain."

Take the case of Edward Gibson. Gibson was known as the Human Pincushion. In his vaudeville act, he would allow audience members to stick pins in him anywhere except his groin and abdomen. During one show, Gibson decided to reenact the Crucifixion, and a woman in the audience fainted when a man with a sledgehammer drove the first spike into Gibson's left hand. At that point, he wisely decided to cancel the show.

Edward Gibson likely had a congenital insensitivity to pain. This condition is part of a spectrum of hereditary neuropathies. People may experience altered pain and/or temperature sensations. They may have problems with regulating their blood pressure or excessive sweating (these functions are controlled by a part of the body called the autonomic nervous system, which may be affected by some neuropathies).

A major problem in people with congenital insensitivity to pain is their inability to protect their bodies. For example, a young boy in the Netherlands who had this condition suffered a series of minor injuries that ultimately led to the collapse and dislocation of both of his hips.

Congenital insensitivity to pain has led researchers to believe that there is tremendous survival value in experiencing pain. What happens every time we sit too long in the same position or we step into a shower that is too hot? We move. We protect our bodies.

Our pain tells us things about our bodies that we need to pay attention to. I call this listening to the voice of your body. Your pain is talking to you. What is it telling you? Whatever your pain is saying (whether it's whispering or shouting), share this with your doctor, because he or she can't hear it—only you can.

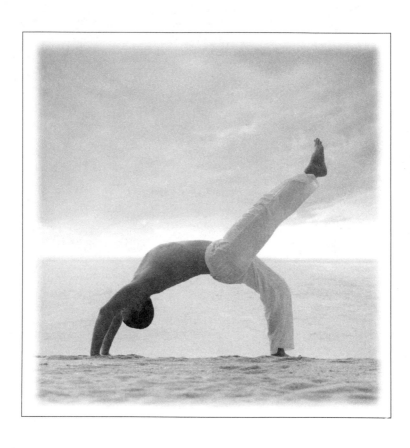

Chapter 4
I Can't Live Like This

Teacher Bag Syndrome

Always laden with books, student assignments, projects and other treasures from my day in the classroom, I would lug my teacher bag home on a daily basis. It was a necessary companion because, as a teacher, my work was never done.

After years of this daily ritual, a dull, aching pain surfaced in my upper back, near my right shoulder blade. The discomfort slowly worsened as the years passed, eventually becoming a constant ache and annoyance. My back pain had become a way of life.

Feeling pity for me, my twenty-seven-year-old daughter, Dana, volunteered to massage my back. Nothing had ever hurt so bad or felt so good at the same time. As she rubbed my back, she was aghast at the knots she could feel in my tightened muscles. "Momma, this is terrible. You need to see a doctor." And, then it was over. Her wonderful three-minute massage had come to an end. My temporary escape into paradise had come to an abrupt halt.

Occasionally, she would agree to rub my back again, but in time, I became a nuisance to her, always begging and pleading for a massage. Eventually, I quit imposing.

By now, I had retired and was no longer a slave to my

teacher bag. My daily travel companion and I finally parted ways. But, our years together had taken a toll on me. The pain in my back now extended up to my shoulder and down my right arm. My pain had become so severe that I could barely lift my arm and I was losing muscle strength. Easy household tasks were becoming difficult for me, if not impossible. But, I persevered as bravely as possible, although complaining excessively.

"Oh! It hurts!" became my endless motto. Not that voicing my discomfort helped, but it just seemed necessary.

My husband, Bob, finally gave me an ultimatum. "Go to the doctor or stop complaining." He was drained of empathy. Enough was enough. So, I made an appointment.

"How long have you had this pain?" Dr. Kinsey inquired, as she flipped through my chart. "About fifteen years," I sheepishly responded. She quickly looked up from my chart in a questioning manner, her gaze lasting uncomfortably long. "I have teacher bag syndrome," I conjectured, admitting that carrying a heavy bag home every day for thirty-two years wasn't such a good practice, at least not for my back, shoulder, and arm.

Steroids and physical therapy were prescribed. Neither turned out to be my friend. The steroids helped with muscle inflammation, but kept me awake for days, and created emotional havoc in my life and in the lives of anyone in my presence. Needless to say, I was elated when my last pill was swallowed and steroid therapy ended.

In physical therapy, I was shuffled between therapists and therapists-in-training. No one followed my case closely to monitor improvement. Their prescription for me was to strengthen muscles in my back, shoulder, and arm through exercise, and they rarely wavered from that order. "I need you to massage the muscles in my back," I would plead. Several of the therapists would occasionally honor that request. Others flatly refused, explaining that was not included in my prescription. When my sessions ended, my back still hurt and I was becoming despondent. Would I suffer this back pain for the rest of my life?

Then, on Mother's Day, my older daughter, Kristen, gave me a gift certificate for a massage. I had never had a professional massage, so I was a bit intimidated by the gesture and held onto the certificate for months before redeeming it. But, as the pain worsened, I finally called for an appointment.

The receptionist recommended a young man for my deep tissue massage. I promptly declined, explaining this was my first massage and, no, it wouldn't be with a man. Laughing softly, she chose another therapist, and my appointment was set with Katie.

Katie was an attractive young woman in her twenties. Her demeanor was pleasant, and my nervousness began subsiding as she accompanied me to the massage room. She listened attentively as I explained my pain issues, and with confidence, assured me I would feel better after our session.

After I had positioned myself face down on the massage table, per Katie's instructions, she returned to the room and the massage of a lifetime began. Pain never felt so good. She massaged and massaged and massaged my painful back, neck, shoulders and arms. After an hour, when the massage was complete, I literally could not move. It was as if I had been massaged into the table. Finally, I managed to roll myself off the table and get dressed, attempting to regain some semblance of reality. My back, shoulders, and arm muscles had never known such painful joy. My muscles and I were on a natural high.

As I was leaving the massage clinic, the young receptionist persuaded me to join their club for monthly massages. She knew I was an easy mark. She knew I would be back.

With ongoing massages, my pain has finally diminished from its previous level of intensity. The pain I feel now is bearable. Katie and I have nine months of massage therapy behind us and there continues to be progress with each visit.

Since my goal is to eventually be pain-free, I will continue my massage therapy as long as it takes. I am now able to raise my arm, my shoulder and back hurt less, and the strength has returned to muscles that lay dormant during my painful years. For me, that feels great! For Katie, well... that's job security.

— Brenda Cook —

The Real Deal

I remember the words he spoke as a tear welled up in my eye. "Well Carissa," he raised his brows, took in a breath and let out an almost scripted sigh. "What can I say; you're just the real deal."

The real deal? As opposed to what? The fake deal? And where's my "real" doctor anyway? Since when is it okay for a physician's assistant to tell a patient that she's in need of surgery? I suppose he was trying to be empathetic. After all, this was my seventh surgery in seven years.

My head was starting to spin. I held back my frustration. And who is "Carissa" anyway? It's Carisa, buddy! Ca-Ree-Sa! You would think after all we've been through he would surely know how to pronounce my name. After all he has seen almost as much of my body as my husband has. With his words gently fading in and out I stared blankly around the tiny six by nine foot office. It smelled of hospital sanitizer and floral perfume, probably from the last patient who was told of her painful fate.

"Here are your prescriptions for preoperative blood work, an EKG, your LSO corset, a CT scan and a lumbar myelogram. Remember, bring your CT scan and myelogram disc on surgery day or we will have to reschedule the whole thing." He paused and fell silent. "Carissa, are you listening?"

His words startled me out of my dejected trance. I adjusted

myself on the table and tore the paper covering as I moved. The wrinkled sheet of paper was sticking to the back of my leg.

"Oops. Sorry, Sam." Yes, the P.A. and I were on a first name basis by then, except he still couldn't or wouldn't pronounce my name correctly, even after seven years.

"I'm still listening. Blood work, EKG, CT, myelogram, brace. Got it."

Gosh, another three months in that giant turtle shell of a brace. I dreaded it. It was my twin sister's daughter Julia, who was two at the time of my first lumber fusion, who coined the now synonymous term "turtle shell." It made me laugh so hard when she asked why I was wearing one. I couldn't explain that it was an LSO corset brace and why I needed it. So, when just three years and five lumbar surgeries later my younger sister's children, four-year-old Luke and two-year-old Ava saw it again, I stuck with it. "You can color Aunt Carisa's turtle shell if you want, but be careful because Aunt Carisa has a big boo-boo under there." Surprisingly, they became very protective of me and my "big boo-boos" over the years.

"We need to get you into surgery in two weeks." Again his voice interrupted my reverie.

I know I was acting like an overgrown child, daydreaming while the teacher was lecturing the class, but I knew the drill by now, and to me it was like riding a bike. After 38 neurosurgery appointments, 20 orthopedic surgeon visits, 8 lumbar myelograms, 17 MRIs, 9 CT scans, 7 lumbar laminectomy surgeries, 3 lumbar fusions, using a walker at age thirty, needing a buggy to ride around the grocery store, a spine built of titanium rods and screws, and seven years of my new married life spent in and out of the hospital, this bionic woman was a pro.

I guess it sounds like I carry a lot of anger and resentment around with me, but truthfully it is the exact opposite. Using humor to get through my tedious doctor appointments has helped me. It's become my coping mechanism. So, a silly thought here and there in a stressful situation couldn't possibly hurt. I really am always listening. After all this is my health we're talking about. Crazy, but true, that I went through the five stages of grief and held pity parties in my honor after my first two visits with the operating table.

I needed a swift kick in the pants to get me out of my slump. It was my husband and best friend Ralph, the love of my life, who nursed me back to health after each traumatic operation that reminded me, no matter how many surgeries I had or may need again, he would always be there. "You are still as beautiful as the day we met fifteen years ago." His words always helped heal me.

So now, at thirty-seven years old, and four months out of my seventh lumber surgery, heading to my eighth, things have gotten better. Sometimes, I can walk on my own without my cane. Medication and my trusty heat pad help when the pain in my legs and back becomes unbearable, and it gets better. It's in those better times that you need to live life. You may have to adjust the way you do things, and for me it's been a constant learning experience. Where's the closest pillow? How long will I need to sit?

I make sure I get plenty of rest. You always heal on the

outside first, so you have to take it easy because you can't see what's going on inside. I have these relentless talks with myself. My degenerative disc disease isn't curable, but I've learned I can fight it. When you have people who love you, your family, in your corner of the proverbial boxing ring picking you up when you are facing another T.K.O. maybe someday you can really "Say Goodbye to Back Pain!" forever. Until then, I guess he was right, I'm just the real deal.

~ Carisa J. Burrows ~

Back to Me

I went down like a brick right after I grabbed for my morning cup of coffee. The pain sheared through not only my back and legs but through the core of my spirit. It was searing, like white-hot electricity, and like nothing I had ever felt before. I had been bothered with flare-ups for the past fifteen years, but this was different. Thankfully my husband was home that day to call for an ambulance, because I had "fallen and couldn't get up."

The first thing they did when I got to the hospital was schedule an MRI for me. The dark, narrow tunnel that enveloped me for almost an hour was like a tomb that would come to symbolize the end of one life and also the womb that would give birth to a new life. "You fractured a disk," the surgeon said. "You're going to need back surgery." He said it the same way my butcher says I need to try the veal. He was so nonchalant that it took me a moment to understand what he was saying.

My super busy life flashed before my eyes: my business, my family, my friends, my home and my pets. But I reassured myself. "I'll be fine. I'm healthy and in good shape. I walk three miles every morning before I go to work in my hair salon. I'm always on the move." I believed that someone in such great shape would do well after surgery. And most importantly, people depended on me. My clients needed me. My husband needed me. My parents needed me. My friends needed me.

But what I wouldn't realize, until years later, is that I needed me. My life had become so out of balance that my body had to break to get my attention. Furthermore, my body wouldn't recover after the surgery.

It's called "failed back surgery." I wasn't sure if I failed or the doctor did, but that didn't matter because I had to try and figure out what kind of life I could make for myself while spending most of the first three years after the surgery bed-ridden. I couldn't stand, sit, or walk for more than five or ten minutes at a time. All I was able to do, for those first few years, was think and pray, and if I was lucky and had a good day, dress myself and make dinner for my husband. "What good am I like this?" I asked anyone in earshot. "Maybe you could use me as a doorstop because I'm not good for anything else."

The emotional suffering of not being able to do my normal daily tasks was unbearable. I had to give up my business as well as anything else from my previous life. I couldn't be depended on by anyone and that was the hardest part. I had gone from being very active and social to being alone most of the time, with no one to listen to but myself. So, I started to write my thoughts in a journal.

Everyone always told me that I was a good listener, but I realized I had listened to so many other voices that I could no longer hear my own. That is until I started journaling. Writing opened a channel within me that allowed me to hear my own truth, to hear what I needed. After losing so much of who I was, or thought I was, writing gave me a new freedom and sovereignty that I hadn't know before. Struggling with unrelenting pain made me feel powerless, but reading the words I had written gave me back a stronger sense of me—of who and all that I was, even though my body was being assaulted by pain.

I would start my journal's pages with things like:

My purpose is...

I have learned...

I trust in...

I have no limits because...

And then I wrote until I exhausted all possibilities. This is where my healing began. It didn't matter that I had lost most of my physical abilities, because I was onto something new—a new way of thinking, a new way of "moving." What used to be merely a physical experience was soon becoming much deeper, more meaningful, and divinely insightful. Before my surgery, I lived out of habit, playing the role of a woman on the move, never having time to go within and give thought to anything other than what I was doing at the time. I was completely out of balance. Running from one thing to the next, for everyone else, left me depleted of my own life force; I was out of gas and broken down. It's no wonder I ended up with chronic pain. While at a pain clinic, a nurse once told me, "People with chronic pain tend to think more of others than they do of themselves. It's a balance issue and something has to give. You need to be there for yourself first."

Journaling was a gift I gave myself. I had read studies about how it can help ease chronic pain, clarify your priorities, and even boost your immune system, but I didn't believe it until I experienced it firsthand. My journal has become my counselor, my friend, and my savior. It's the wisest voice I hear. It keeps me in check and in touch with what I'm feeling. I can tell when I'm out of balance by what I'm writing. I can tell when I'm pressured and when I'm pushing myself too hard. I know that when I get stressed, it's usually a precursor to a flare-up, which I can see coming through the written thoughts I pour onto the page.

I always had carried the weight of the world on my back. I felt that I was on call, so to speak, for everyone else. There are still days when I struggle with that mindset, but I understand now that I need to show up for my own life. I have to slow down and pay attention to my needs, because it's truly the only way I can be there for others. Writing in my journal shows me how to do that, in the most surprising ways!

— Marijo Herndon —

What If
It Works?

"I don't want to mess with physical therapy," I said.

My neurosurgeon crossed his legs and folded his hands to listen. "Why not?"

I leaned against the exam table and shifted my weight. As I did, the paper table cover crinkled. I couldn't sit down. The pain from a line-up of bulging and protruding disks was too great. "Doctor, I don't have time. Therapy will take weeks and weeks, and may not even work. I have five children at home. I crawl from room to room, to wake them in the mornings." I bit my lip to keep from crying. "I can't care for my family from the floor. It's that simple. I want to have surgery again. It's faster."

I wasn't minimizing the significance of surgery. The risks. The recovery time. The pain. I'd gone that route before. But right now I needed to be moving forward. In the most soon-as-possible way. Five days a week, indefinitely, for therapy, didn't seem to be the most expedient route. If only the doctor would understand that I'd lain on the bathroom floor that morning, trying to dry my toddler after he'd hurled himself in and out of the bathtub.

"Surgery is invasive and a last resort. I want you to try therapy first. I'll have Sandy call the therapy center. We'll get you scheduled."

"What if it doesn't work?" I asked. I imagined my family needing their mama. If it didn't work, it would have been a waste of time. Time that I didn't have. My family had needs that a pain-racked, nearly immobile mama couldn't address.

My surgeon's chair creaked as he leaned back and crossed his arms. "Well, what if it does?"

I was scheduled for my first therapy appointment the next morning. Lonny, my husband, took the day off from work to drive me. I couldn't sit upright. I stretched across the middle seat of our Suburban, bobbing and rolling and wincing with each bump. He helped me from the truck and inched me through the heavy July air. By the time the cold blast of office air hit my face, I was angry. Red-hot pain from that disk shot down my leg. And I hated feeling helpless, wanting to sit down to wait but standing by the coat rack instead.

"Wish I could've been scheduled for surgery today," I whispered into Lonny's ear. "Last time, the day after surgery, the pain was gone. It was all uphill from there."

Lonny smiled a sympathetic smile and rooted through his wallet for his insurance card.

I whispered a little louder. "I don't want to mess with this."

Just then a tall, well muscled man called my name. He stood in the doorway with a clipboard and a smile. "My name is Mark," he said, as I inched toward him. He offered his strong, warm hand.

Mark led us to an exam room. For the longest time, he allowed me to talk. About my back. About the pain. About my need to care for my family and my desire to hold my boys on my lap and toss them Nerf balls and prepare their meals and turn down their beds. I shared about my surgical experience and recovery and the fresh, debilitating experience with pain. Then Mark did an exam and measured my mobility, which I later learned, was limited to an extreme.

"Before we work on a treatment plan," Mark said, as I stood in the corner of the tiny room, "we need to get your back in alignment. We'll start by having you lie prostrate." Mark looked at my husband. "Lonny, I'll show you how to lift her hips to straighten her out."

I reluctantly eased myself to the table, and with the help of the two men, rolled to my tummy.

"Her back looks like an S," Lonny said.

Mark didn't say a word. He just showed Lonny how to gently lift my hips to align them with my shoulders. "This will take pressure off the disks," he said. "You'll need to be this way for twenty minutes every hour."

He also shared that chairs were off-limits. I pictured my family around the table without me.

Hot tears slipped from my eyes. But they didn't have far to fall. I was already face down.

The sun shone high and bright in the midday sky the next day. But I felt dark inside. I had an appointment with Mark, and I'd spent a great deal of time sprawled on the floor while my family bustled around me. "Mama." Isaiah, my toddler, lifted his arms to me as I shuffled toward the door.

"Mama can't lift you, Zay," I said. "But I love you. So much."

No. This prolonged treatment was not going to work.

"How is your pain today?" Mark asked, first thing. He sat across from me, clipboard in hand.

"It's a smidgen better."

"Good. Let's measure your mobility."

Mark and I worked through what would become the daily routine. Questions. Measurements. And eventually stretching and exercise. I was a passive participant. Mark moved my legs. One day he introduced an electrotherapy device. A great belt with straps the next. Each day I was given "homework." Standing against the wall with a pillow wedged under my shoulder. Prostrate on the ground with my elbows propped. I scheduled my appointments a week at a time, and the days passed like molasses.

One afternoon the whole family came for my appointment. It was double-dip ice cream day at the local ice cream shop, and we wanted to treat the boys. My family waited in the reception area as I went to the exam room for an appointment with Mark.

I sat on the table and waited for his questions.

"How is the pain when you sit?" he asked.

Sit? I hadn't even thought about it. But I'd walked into that room and had sat down! I hadn't been at the table with my family for weeks, and there I was, sitting, without much pain.

"Not so bad," I said.

"Very, very good," Mark said.

I was smiling as he and I went through the normal routine of exercise. At the end of our session, he told me that I was ready to move to the exercise room for active therapy.

"I'm making progress," I said, a feeling of hope taking root in my heart.

"You're doing very, very well," Mark said.

At the end of our session, I went to the reception area to meet my family. My youngest son took my hand. "Can you get some ice cream, too, Mama?"

I squeezed his palm against mine. "Yes! I think I can."

My therapy sessions continued. Mark was knowledgeable, supportive, and strong. He'd gained my trust, and I felt safe in his care.

Six weeks after my therapy began, Mark gave me my "walking papers." How appropriate, as I walked, with full mobility, out that office door. My family had managed just fine, and I was recovered and ready to resume my life full-force.

I often think back to my doctor's response when I questioned therapy. "What if it doesn't work?" I'd asked.

His answer was simple.

"Well, what if it does?"

— Shawnelle Eliasen —

I Can't Live Like This

Brenda's story about her "teacher bag syndrome" is one I've heard many times by patients coming in for neck and mid-back pain. Sometimes a heavy bag will also affect the low back (since your spine and all of the nerves, muscles, tendons, and ligaments connect in some way to each other). There are many variations on this story that I hear from carpenters (who carry tools and wear tool belts), business people (who carry briefcases and/or suitcases when they travel), teenagers (who carry backpacks) and so on. What made Brenda finally seek help for her pain after fifteen years? There were likely multiple factors, including that she was now retired and had more time to focus on herself. But, probably the single most important thing that caused her to seek help was that she thought, "I can't live like this!"

When I hear a story like Brenda's, I'm always wondering whether the patient sitting in front of me has an official diagnosis. Then, my next thought is, "Does she have the *right* diagnosis?" In Brenda's case, it's hard to tell the answer to either question. Teacher bag syndrome is not a medical diagnosis. Sure, heavy bags can cause problems, but what is actually her diagnosis? And, is it the right one? (She might have a formal diagnosis for her back pain that she didn't mention in her story.) Here's what I'd be thinking if Brenda were in my office:

1. Do you have a diagnosis?

2. Do you have the right diagnosis?
3. Have you seen a doctor?
4. Have you seen the right doctor for your condition?
5. Have you had any tests to diagnose your condition?
6. Have you had the right tests to diagnose your condition?
7. Have you tried any treatment?
8. Have you tried the right treatment for your condition?

Back pain — whether it's in the upper, mid or lower region — can be difficult to diagnose because there are so many structures that could be injured and causing pain. However, before I recommend any medical treatment, I must first decide what I think the diagnosis is, or at least what I think the most likely diagnosis is.

In a nutshell, here's why some people have chronic back pain without significant relief of their symptoms: They've never been properly diagnosed, and the treatment interventions they've tried are not targeted for their particular diagnosis.

Even though this is true, and I want to emphasize how important it is to try and figure out the right diagnosis, it's not always possible to do so. Our backs have so many complicated structures that may play a role in pain that there are times when it's challenging to figure out what is causing discomfort. Even with excellent physicians and state-of-the-art testing, it's not always possible to solve the diagnosis dilemma. Nevertheless, if you are living with back pain, and you want some relief, keep this in mind: Finding the right diagnosis may be the key to getting targeted treatment that really works.

Who Is on Your Team?

Often people see more than one type of practitioner to alleviate back pain, starting with a generalist and then seeking more specific types of help. Here's a quick guide to the type of clinicians you might encounter.

Physicians

Primary care physician: Trained in general medicine, internal medicine, or family practice; makes referrals to specialists as necessary.

Neurologist: Focuses on treatment of the nerves and nervous system.

Neurosurgeon: Provides surgical care of nerve-related problems.

Orthopedist: Diagnoses and treats problems of the skeletal system and its muscles, joints and ligaments. Some orthopedists also perform spine surgeries.

Osteopath: Has training similar to that of an M.D. Osteopaths utilize some treatment modalities that most M.D.'s are not trained to do such as spinal manipulation.

Physiatrist: Rehabilitation physician that specializes in musculoskeletal medicine, including non-surgical or post-surgical back problems.

Rheumatologist: Specializes in the treatment of rheumatic diseases (those affecting the joints, muscles, bones, skin and other tissues), some of which can affect the back.

Other professionals

Chiropractor: Trained in manipulation of the bones and joints, including those in the spine.

Physical therapist: Focuses on exercises and other rehabilitative techniques to restore function and mobility.

Occupational therapist: Focuses on workstation evaluations, posture, adaptive equipment and upper body strength and range of motion.

Massage Therapist: May help with decreasing muscle stress and tension.

Acupuncturist: Some pain conditions will respond to acupuncture.

Do I Have Sciatica?

Many of my patients tell me, "My doctor sent me to you because I have sciatica." Sometimes this is true, but more often than not, they don't actually have sciatica. At least, they don't have injury to the sciatic nerve.

Medical dictionaries often define "sciatica" as severe pain in the leg along the course of the sciatic nerve, typically felt at the back of the thigh and calf. Of course this implies, and most people believe, that the sciatic nerve is the source of the problem. However, the symptoms associated with this type of pain are not usually due to injury to the sciatic nerve.

The sciatic nerve is the biggest nerve in the body and arises below the level of the spine in a big grouping of nerves called the sacral plexus. Specific injury to the sciatic nerve is actually not all that common. The most common cause of "sciatica" is actually a condition called lumbosacral radiculopathy. Frequently this is due to a herniated disk in the spine (above the level of the sciatic nerve) that is pressing on a nerve that supplies the muscles to the leg (for example, the L5 or S1 nerve root—which is the 5th lumbar or 1st sacral spinal nerve root).

Sciatica is a term that people may use to describe back and leg pain (sometimes associated with burning, numbness and/or tingling), rather than an actual diagnosis.

Though the real diagnosis still exists, it's just not all that common.

So, if you think you have sciatica, ask your doctor whether you really might have a lumbar or sacral (lumbosacral for short) radiculopathy. The treatment for radiculopathy is not the same as it would be for injury to the sciatic nerve. Treating the wrong diagnosis usually means that people don't get better.

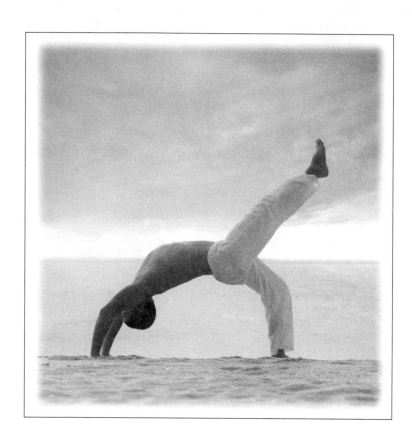

Chapter 5
Life Is
Stressful

My Husband's Motto

Police Chief Eddie R. Defew found himself in numerous dangerous situations during his twenty-five years of public service. For instance, once he stopped a man for reckless driving when he swerved into a funeral possession, nearly hitting another vehicle. After finding out the man was intoxicated, he reached through the man's driver side window to remove his keys from the ignition. That's when the man took off, dragging Eddie for several yards down the street. Thinking fast, he kicked away from the moving truck to prevent being run over by a rear tire and was thrown loose.

When he got up and brushed himself off, he knew he was scraped and sore, but didn't think he was seriously hurt. A few days later, he could barely turn his head without excruciating stabs of pain. His doctor could find nothing wrong, so Eddie chalked it up to normal hazardous duty like his job description read. Over the years, he had his share of near misses, but the neck pain from that one particular day never went away.

In the fall of 1988, while on vacation from his job, he went hunting with a friend. At sundown, the two hunters came back to the truck to pack up and start home. As his friend unloaded his rifle, it accidentally went off, hitting Eddie in the shoulder and chest. After twenty-eight days in the hospital, the doctor who saved his arm and his life said, "Ten out of ten men would have died. You shouldn't have lived." But, he warned him about the pain he would have in the future. "You'll know when a weather change is coming long before the weather man does."

The doctor was right. Along with the shoulder and neck pain, in 1994 he was diagnosed with degenerative arthritis of the spine, a pain that radiated up and down his spine. The cushioning between his vertebrae was disappearing, causing them to rub bone against bone, adding more pain to his collection of injuries.

In 1994, I met Eddie. He had retired and was looking forward to a simpler, more peaceful life. That sounded good to me. For ten years, I had fought rheumatoid arthritis and its crippling effects while trying to work a full-time job. We had a lot in common. Each of us had been divorced for several years and had experienced our fair share of pain, both physical and mental. As fate would have it, we hit it off, married two years later, and moved to his farm in the country. Even with our underlying health problems, we had never been happier.

Then, ten years later, while deer hunting, Eddie felt an excruciating pain run down his back. For days, he could hardly walk or drive. He tried to describe it to his doctor, "It feels like your hand feels when you've laid on it at night and, when it comes to life, it feels like a thousand needles prickling your skin." Only, with him, the episodes went on non-stop for hours at a time. "It feels like I'm holding my foot in freezing cold water," he explains. "But, it's not cold to the touch. In fact, if the pain is really intense, my leg actually sweats." A lifelong jogger, the weakening muscles in his left leg worried him a lot too.

After a series of CT scans, the doctor found the primary reason for his pain. It was coming from the L3/L4 section of his spine. One disc was bulging; one disc was herniated. As a result, his sciatic nerve was being pinched, causing the pain in his left leg and foot. "I can send you to a specialist," he offered. "Surgery is an option, but there are no guarantees." Eddie's damage was so extensive, surgery could actually make it worse instead of better.

So, after careful consideration, Eddie decided to take the road that made more sense to him. "If worse comes to worse, I'll see a surgeon. But, until that day, I'll take it a day at a time and hope the days stretch into years." From that point on, he began an exercise regime to strengthen his lower back muscles and he gradually got back to his normal routine of jogging. Instead of giving in to the pain, he would learn to live with it.

Our farm was the motivating factor. He loved it with all his heart. "When we moved to the country," he said, "I felt like I'd finally come home." I felt the same, but it did include lots of chores and responsibilities. Although I would do all I could to help, I was limited by my disease. I wondered if he would be able to keep it up.

I should have known better. My husband's not one to give up on something he loves. When it comes to the pain, there's never a day that he doesn't fight back. I often ask him how he does it when I see him refuse to give in. "If I'm busy," he says, "I don't think so much about the pain. And, if I sit down, I might not ever get up." So, instead of slowing down, he pushes himself even more, a mind-over-matter approach that works for him. When the job is done, he may be exhausted from fighting the pain, but he feels good about himself.

So, to make sure he keeps on moving forward, Eddie starts a new project every year, doing something he's always wanted to do. So far, with the help of some very good friends, he has managed to build a cabin with a dock on our pond, a man-cave in the barn where all his buddies gather, a cookout shelter to house a barbecue pit, a chicken house for our eight chickens, dog kennels for our five kennel dogs, an authentic chuck wagon for Dutch oven cooking, and an old log cabin for a guest house. He has also planted gardens fit for a magazine cover and planted acres of food plots for the wildlife. His plate is always full.

And, his perseverance is contagious. Once people see him creating and constructing, they are inspired to jump in and be part of it. No matter what their own health obstacles may be, he pushes them to follow his lead. His tenacity inspires others to face life's challenges, to become part of the solution rather than the problem. However, he is quick to say he expects no more of them than he does of himself.

It's a busy life filled with many blessings in the form of family, friends, and our beloved dogs. For us, staying busy is a powerful remedy for ignoring pain. But, when there's no one else around and pain shows its relentless head, we rely on one another to keep going. Just knowing we are there for each other makes all the difference. In the meanwhile, I've become a firm believer in my husband's motto: "I'm going to keep on working the best I can, for as long as I can. The pain will just have to get used to it."

— Linda C. Defew —

Simple Changes

Oh, that hurt! I held my breath as I attempted to roll from my back onto my side. I had always been strong and active. I contemplated the pain that ran from my right hip down the front of my leg as I lay in bed. I could understand back pain during everyday activities or overexertion, but trying to turn from my back onto my side while lying down?

I stretched regularly and received an occasional massage. I had gone to physical therapy and to a chiropractor and I took an occasional anti-inflammatory. What else was there? How many avenues could I pursue? I hated exercise.

My responsibilities are physically demanding. I have a large house, property and animals that take more time than there is in a day. That day, as I lifted six fifty-pound bags of animal feed onto the bed of the truck I wondered who would take care of all of this if something happened to me. And then I noticed my upper back and shoulders tightening and my teeth slightly clenching as I turned to walk up the rolling hills that led to the garden. As always, I felt like I had to hurry. I needed to get the gardening done before it got too hot.

Maybe that tension and stress explained the knot between my shoulders, my neck pain and the headaches. I started to analyze my activities. If my muscles were weak, they couldn't support my body when I leaned forward to climb that hill to the garden. The tendons tightened and tried to compensate. This created tension. I needed to strengthen the weak muscles and stretch the strong ones. My body needed to be balanced. Tension was also restricting blood and fluid that was needed by my spine to keep discs healthy.

Walking up another incline I took a deep breath, only this time I relaxed my shoulders, exhaled and dropped my weight into my hands. Standing tall, I felt my shoulders stretch and my neck relax. I decided to make a conscious effort to recognize and eliminate tension, starting that day.

As I started to cultivate my small garden with a hoe, I realized that the right side of my body was doing all of the work. I led with my right foot. My right arm and hand were in charge. My left was mainly for support. I could feel something pulling in my right hip and lower back. That was it! That was the same place I felt the pain when I tried to turn over in bed. I remembered what a massage therapist had told me at one point: "Repeated activities using one side of your body will cause your body to become unbalanced. Use both sides of your body." I am so right-sided it's ridiculous, but I decided to give it a try.

So, I rotated my body, taking my right foot back and leading with my left. Switching my hands around, I started to hoe weeds with my left hand and used my right for balance. It was awkward and much slower. It was not the most efficient way to tend a garden as I chopped at the ground between the rows of vegetables. As I chopped, I occasionally missed my target. I wondered what the penalty was for murdering carrots.

Day after day I tried to perform everyday chores with the

left side of my body as well as my dominant right side. It became easier over time and the benefits were worth the effort. Within a couple of weeks after I started my new routine, I noticed that there was less pain. A short time later I turned from my back onto my side. Then I realized... the pain was gone!

~ Paula Naughton ~

Fit to Be Tied

With a sigh, I picked up the sports magazine from the shelf in the waiting room. Over the years, I had delighted in playing volleyball and badminton. I swam in the college pool three times a week. I biked and walked regularly. Free weights, an exercise ball and stretch bands at home were my routine on days when rain or snow prevented outdoor exercise. Yet here I was at the physical therapist's office again.

Sure, some of my previous visits related to sports injuries. I gave up swinging a badminton racket after undergoing a year of therapy for tennis elbow, but I continued to play in the fifty-five-plus volleyball league—my team went to nationals my final year of competitive play. Then I had torn a hamstring, sprained an ankle, damaged the miniscus in first one knee and then the other, and strained my rotator cuff. The hard reality was that diving for wild balls, tossing up hard serves and jumping to spike a ball over the net were joys of the past. I gave up playing and resigned myself to watching my children compete on their college teams. Each new injury I faced limited my options for an active lifestyle. Now my back was causing problems.

Would I have to give up one more activity? If so, how would I stay in shape? I fumed. I felt frustrated. I was fit to be tied.

Much as I appreciated Mandy, my physical therapist, I had no desire to spend any more time at her office. Yet here I was at her office again. When I rose each morning, pain radiated from my spine down into my left hip. Every step I took activated an acute jab that forced me to gasp. I could no longer stand at the sink washing dishes. Leaning over to do a simple task such as emptying the dishwasher or unloading the clothes dryer resulted in unrelenting pain.

Previous experience had made me wary of X-rays and MRI studies. Nothing of consequence ever showed up. This time, rather than go that route, I had decided to begin where I always ended up, at Mandy's office.

"So what are we in for today?" Mandy led me into the small spare room with an examination table.

I handed her the forms the receptionist had given me to fill out. On the small illustration of a person I had drawn arrows to my hip and symbols indicating the type of pain. Another portion of the chart indicated my level of pain and how it impacted my daily activities. Suddenly the enormity of fighting pain for many years on a daily basis overwhelmed me. Tears began to roll down my cheeks.

Embarrassed, I mopped up with a towel and struggled to control my emotions. "It just seems that one thing after another falls apart. It is so discouraging. I try to stay in shape. After doing all the exercises you have given me, I still have pain."

Part physical therapist and part counselor, Mandy nodded her head. When I was calmer, she asked me to bend forward and backward while she observed. Then, placing me on the examining table, she stretched me to the left and the right. She took measurements and asked more questions. As always her thoroughness impressed me. She confirmed that the hip pain stemmed from a problem in my lower back.

Over the next weeks, Mandy taught me to do push-ups in

a way that arched my lower back and forced spinal disks into proper alignment. She worked on strengthening my core to support the weak area of my spine. She always amazed me when she could find one more way to stretch a muscle I didn't know I had. Thankfully, through it all I was able to continue swimming. The buoyancy of the water offered a brief respite from my daily pain.

One day, as I watched, Mandy introduced yet another new exercise. To demonstrate it, she lay down on her back on the examining table. Lifting and bending her right leg in the air, she raised and bent her left leg at ninety degrees to place her ankle in front of the right knee. Then with her arms around her right thigh, she pulled both legs toward her chest. The motion turned her into a human pretzel.

"You're kidding!" I gasped.

She laughed and assured me that she was serious. This exercise stretched the hip flexors. It took some coaching on her part but at last I was able to duplicate the strange feat. The muscles in my hip protested as I pulled them beyond their comfort zone. My limbs were tied in a knot.

More weeks passed. Slowly, surely, the pain subsided as my back grew stronger. The pain never disappeared altogether, but it decreased to a tolerable level. Today my hip only protests at the start of the day. By the time I have spent half an hour at the pool or on the track, my back has settled into place. I faithfully do all of Mandy's exercises, including twisting myself into a human knot. With the help of my physical therapist, I'm once again "fit" to be tied.

— Emily Parke Chase —

An Ironman Triathlon, Really?

I have been suffering from spondylolisthesis ("spondy") at L5 (which is basically a slippage of the vertebrae so they become out of alignment) since I was in high school, but I didn't know it at the time. I was a gymnast for quite a few years until it got to the point where I was in constant back pain and couldn't compete anymore. Those were the days before spring floors! So, I switched to become a cheerleader. In hindsight, this wasn't the best idea because then I was doing gymnastics on hardwood floors instead of on the more cushy mats. But I was a teenager and wasn't thinking about that or any long-term consequences of this decision.

For several years, every few months my back would "go out" on me. I didn't know why. When my back went out, I could not lift my legs without pain that took my breath away. When I was in my early twenties it got so bad that I finally went to a doctor, who diagnosed the spondy. He said that if I did exercises to keep my middle section strong, it would help, but that this condition was chronic and could not be fixed unless I had surgery, which could cause its own problems.

To make it worse, when I was twenty-eight I was showing

my four-year-old daughter a gymnastics move on the playground. When I landed the "trick," my body couldn't remember how to hold the move and I tore my Anterior Crutiate Ligament (ACL). Three months later I re-tore the reconstruction and had a second ACL reconstruction on the same knee. So then I not only had spondy in my lower back, but my strength was lopsided in my legs, which did not bode well for keeping my back in alignment.

In my twenties and thirties, I went to the gym and did some aerobics classes, but did not try to run. In my late thirties the spin craze started and I started to do that two times a week. I thought this might be good for my knee strength. It was in one of those spin classes that the instructor said to me, "Diane, you should join my triathlon training this summer and do a triathlon. I just know you will love it." I thought she was crazy. I hadn't been swimming since I worked at a day camp when I was a teenager. I didn't even own a bicycle. And, I couldn't run more than a mile.

Not to mention, with my back and knee issues, wouldn't I get worse? I was pretty active at the gym and didn't want to jeopardize what exercise I was able to do at the time. After several attempts on her part to recruit me, I finally acquiesced. It sounded like fun. I never really considered myself an athlete, so this would certainly be a challenge.

I embarked on the most amazing journey ever. I started training with her group two times a week and adhering to the training schedule she gave all of us to do when we were not together. I also added core training, which I knew I had to do. But at the time, I really knew nothing about what real core training was.

During this eight-week period, my back would hurt every week, but it didn't completely slip out because I was being very cautious in building up my running distances. I ran as little as I thought would still prepare me for the race. Week after week I got stronger and the prospect of actually finishing a triathlon got more exciting.

Finishing that race was probably one of the hardest things I have ever done, but also one of the most rewarding. I got a taste of athleticism that I never knew I had. I not only completed that sprint distance triathlon but seven more like it over the next year. I caught the bug! But, after each race and training season, I was in a lot of back pain. I decided that if I was going to continue doing triathlons, which I knew I just had to do, I really needed to learn more about how to protect my back.

I read absolutely everything I could on all aspects of training and injury prevention. Along with all the swim/bike/run training, I do lots and lots of core exercises to help protect my back. Within the group that I coach, they have dubbed me the "Core Queen!" Of course, I couldn't do it all by myself. My coaches, physical therapists, massage therapists, orthopedic doctors, chiropractors and acupuncturist all play key parts in keeping me going. They are now collectively and affectionately known as "Team Diane."

I love everything about the process of triathlons—the learning, the training, the racing, and encouraging others to do it. So I decided to become a triathlon coach myself. I started by becoming a workout leader and helping the coach who recruited me. After two years of increasing my knowledge on my own and assisting other coaches, I flew to New Orleans and spent four days in a clinic with USA Triathlon to become a triathlon coach. One of the people I coach has a degenerative back injury. Working with her has been so rewarding.

I never thought that I could progress past the sprint distance triathlons, which are usually a half-mile swim, 12-13 miles on the bike, and a six-mile run. However, as I learned more about strength and core training, I was able to go farther. I actually completed several half marathons and the full Boston Marathon, and also a full iron distance triathlon, several Olympic and half iron distance races as well. Imagine, someone with my physical issues swimming 2.4 miles, riding 112 miles and then running a full marathon, all in the same day!

I still have back pain if I do too much or don't keep up with a core exercise program, but in my mid-forties and nine years after starting triathlons, I'm able to compete in any distance triathlon I want to. I do know that as I get into my fifties and sixties I'll probably need to hang up the longer distance run and triathlon races. But for now, I'll keep doing my core exercises and working with Team Diane to keep my body balanced and my back healthy.

~ Diane Stokes ~

Life Is Stressful

One day a woman came to see me with low back and neck pain due to injuries from a car accident. This woman was obviously in physical pain, but there was more to her story than back pain. She and her husband had been trying to conceive a child for years. Finally, the fertility treatments worked. She was five months pregnant when the accident occurred, and her unborn baby didn't survive.

This is a particularly heartbreaking story, but even when a life isn't lost, it is very common for people to be dealing with a lot more than just back pain. Mandy describes how she began to cry at one of her physical therapy appointments. All health-care providers see patients when they are vulnerable. Physically vulnerable but also emotionally discouraged, frustrated, scared, angry, annoyed or heartbroken. Life can be complicated and extremely stressful. It would be nice to not have other problems to deal with when you are injured and in pain. But, very often it's precisely when you are physically vulnerable that you are also not at your usual emotional baseline.

Cluster Busters

Pain often presents with other symptoms, including difficulty with sleep that causes fatigue, worry that leads to anxiety, frustration that may become depression, and so on. Doctors who treat a lot of pain often look for "cluster symptoms" because they know that treating all of the symptoms at once tends to lead to better outcomes. For example, an 85-year-old-woman who I'll call Joan began to experience pain in her legs when she walked. Prior to having pain, she was very active, though she lived in an assisted living facility. An MRI revealed that her pain was due to lumbar spinal stenosis, a narrowing of the canal at the end of the spine that causes "pinching" of the nerves. Joan tried many different treatments including medications, physical therapy and spinal injections. Nothing was working very well, and she really needed surgery. But I was very hesitant to recommend surgery due to her advanced age.

One day, Joan came in for an appointment, and I changed her medications to try and give her more pain relief. She left and seemed discouraged, but willing to try the change in prescriptions. A few minutes after Joan left, I went to lunch. On my way to lunch, I spotted her sitting alone with her head in her hands weeping. I felt so sad for her and realized that I needed to do more to help her. I went over to her and for the first time she told me about symptoms that she hadn't admitted to me in the office. Joan said that she wasn't sleeping well, because she was stressed and worrying at night. In fact, her anxiety was getting out of control, and she was afraid to leave her room. When she did leave, she worried that she'd have pain and need to find a place to sit down right away. Coupled with insomnia and anxiety, Joan said that she was crying a lot and feeling hopeless — signs of depression. Between her mood problems and lack of sleep, she wasn't concentrating well. Though she was mentally sharp, Joan began to think that she was developing Alzheimer's.

Joan was experiencing cluster symptoms, and each one was making the others worse. They worked together to significantly decrease her quality of life, and her physical and emotional health was spiraling downward. Right then I decided that despite Joan's age, she really needed a surgical consultation. She also would benefit from consulting with her primary care physician about her mood and sleep issues. Ultimately, I talked to her doctors and we worked out a plan where Joan would take a mild sedative at night to help her sleep and then undergo surgery for her back. She began to sleep better, and with a plan in place to help with her pain, Joan's mood improved. Surgery did solve her pain problems, and within a few weeks, she told me that she was "feeling like I did when I was seventy!"

Although I had asked Joan about possible cluster symptoms, she had consistently told me that her back and leg pain was her primary problem. I wish she had told me about her other symptoms, but I know that many patients "tough it out" when it comes to problems with sleep and mood. It's important to recognize how these symptoms work together to make you feel really bad, or alternately if treated appropriately, really good!

Strained Backs, Strained Relationships

The story about Eddie doing one project a year highlights an important strategy that a lot of people with chronic pain use. Instead of giving up what they love to do, they figure out ways to do what they want but still manage their pain. A patient of mine who struggles with pain calls herself the "One A Day Girl." She books one fun thing to do every day. If she tries to do too much, she suffers. So, when a friend calls and invites her to the movies, if she's already scheduled something for that day, she asks if it's possible to see the film on a day when she doesn't have anything else to do. This way, every day my patient has something to look forward to but doesn't overdo it.

Of course, when you have a lot of people counting on you—family and friends—telling them that you can't do things because of pain can put a lot of stress on those relationships. It's not always easy to balance nurturing yourself and others. And, while there may not be an easy solution to either your back pain or the strain it causes on your relationship, there are some strategies that might work to help you and those you care about feel better:

- Start a "choice diet." We all have many opportunities to say "yes" or "no" to things. What is it that you want to do (or not do)? Be selective and not reactive when someone asks you to do something. Is this a good choice for you? Keep in mind that saying "yes" to one thing means saying "no" to whatever else you might do with that time and energy.

- Build your social capital. Social capital is your "wealth" in human and other connections. In general, studies have shown that people who have a lot of social capital are happier and healthier. Think about ways that you can connect with others—via e-mail, phone, letters or face to face contact. One way that people improve their social capital is to get a pet. Dogs, especially, provide a lot of love and support to their owners. Plus, walking your dog gets you out and about, talking to people in your community.

- Pay a gratitude visit. Identify people who you would like to thank for their kindness. Pay it forward and thank them. If you can do this in person, that's ideal. However, there are a lot of ways to communicate if you can't meet. For the thank-you to be as meaningful as possible, try and be specific. What did this person do that you are grateful for and how did it make you feel? Gratitude visits and other positive psychology strategies have been shown to lessen feelings of sadness and worry.

Sex and Your Aching Back

It's not uncommon for backaches to interfere with an individual's lovemaking. Often, people are reluctant to talk with their doctor about how their back pain affects their sexual activity. But if you find that backaches—or fears of reinjuring your back—put a damper on your sex life, ask your doctor for advice.

Sex and Your Aching Back (continued)

Here are a few suggestions that might also be helpful:

- Talk openly with your partner about your concerns.
- Avoid arching your spine backward. Try to keep your spine straight or bent slightly forward.
- When bending forward, be sure to bend your knees. Bending forward while keeping your knees straight puts a lot of pressure on your lower back.
- Avoid lying on your stomach or your back with your legs flat on the bed and extended straight out. If you can, keep your hips flexed to take some pressure off your lower back.
- Try positions that are easier on your back, such as lying on your side with your hips and your knees slightly bent.
- Be judicious and gentle. If your back is bothering you, don't aim for long, vigorous, gymnastic lovemaking.
- Making love in the water — in a pool or hot tub — can take some of the stress off your back, because water is buoyant and offers support.
- Be patient. Don't try to resume sex too soon after having a backache. If you find that your back hurts when you resume sexual activity, wait a few days before trying again.

Reprinted with permission from the Harvard Health Publications Special Health Report: Low Back Pain (2010)

Get Ready, Set, Go—Ouch!!

Have you ever noticed that just when you are looking forward to something, you experience more pain? Sometimes, getting ready is the problem. For example, a relative or friend is coming to visit, and you want your house to shine a bit so you clean more than usual. Or, the holidays are approaching, and you do things that you don't usually do, such as wrap presents, bake or get ready for guests to arrive. Winter can cause a lot of pain from shoveling snow or slips and falls on the ice, but so can spring and fall when people work out in the yard more than usual.

If you've noticed a pattern of having more pain just when you are looking forward to something, think about what you might be doing prior to the event that is contributing to your symptoms. Here are a few hints:

Avoid repetitive tasks that you are unaccustomed to performing. This is the main reason that I see people coming in with seasonal pain or soreness due to spring gardening or fall yard cleanup. Put simply, they do things that they are not used to doing, and in their rush to get tasks done, they push through the initial warning signs of pain until they become very uncomfortable. Keep in mind that the "big pain" may not come until hours after the task is completed (or even the next day or two), but you will usually get early warning signs that your body is becoming uncomfortable.

Listen to your body—or you may pay a price later. Of course you don't have to completely avoid repetitive tasks, but sitting for hours wrapping presents, taking trays out of the oven, bending over to plant flowers, or raking can create the "perfect storm" to develop or worsen back pain. If you have repetitive tasks to do, be sure and take breaks and stretch. Do something else for a little while, then come back to your task later.

Ask your kids to help. If your kids are sitting around playing electronic games or watching TV, get them involved in helping. Not only will it help you avoid an injury, but it's good for their health.

Get enough sleep. Cutting back on sleep when you are busy puts your body at risk for injuries. Be sure that you are getting enough sleep so that you can enjoy whatever it is that you are looking forward to.

Build fun into your schedule. Chores and "to do" lists should not be the sum total of your day—even before a big event. Be sure and add something fun to your "to do" list. Laugh and enjoy yourself. There is no better time than now!

Find ways to relax. Even when you have a lot to do, find ways to relax. You can meditate, pray, take a long walk, listen to soft music, take a hot bath or do whatever you enjoy that helps calm your mind and ease the stress on your body.

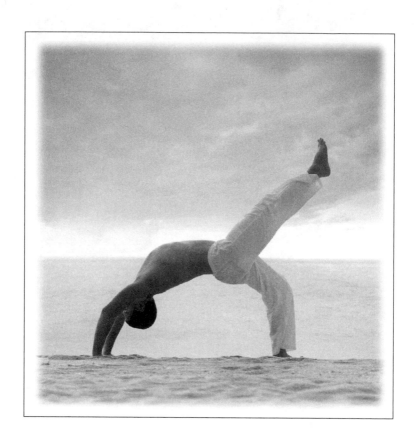

Chapter 6
Finally, Help Is on the Way!

Don't Act
Twenty-One
When You're Not!

Thirty-four years ago, I headed into my younger son's bedroom to wake him before I went to work. As I bent down I sneezed and threw out my back. I could barely return to my bed and crawl in. Pain, spasms, and extreme discomfort hit so fast, it seemed as though I'd been struck by lightning.

My wife called our doctor, who prescribed ice for the first day and then heat, a muscle relaxer, and something for pain. An appointment was made for three days later. I fumed at the wait. I was bullheaded, impatient, and I didn't understand why I had to wait. I was dying. I should have been seen immediately.

By my appointment time, I was able to drive myself to the doctor's office. On a scale of one to ten, my pain had dropped from an eleven to a four. My doctor asked me to do various body poses and walking tasks. After his examination, he said, "My bet is you have a slipped disk caused by the sneeze happening when you were in the wrong position. At your age, I'm guessing time, exercise, and common sense will help you heal."

I took the exercise pamphlet he handed me, grumbled about the common sense comment, and didn't want to hear about letting time take care of things. But I was a young man of thirty-five back then. The pain did go away, and I went on with life as normal.

Five years later, I was on a business trip to Seminole, Texas, with its oil fields, cotton, and dust. My business partner and I had just jumped back into our rental car for the drive to the airport in Midland-Odessa, when I reached into the back seat of the car to pull something out of my briefcase. Bam! My back stabbed me like I'd fallen on a spike.

By then I had a new doctor. But the advice and the medication were the same. Even the list of exercises looked strangely familiar. I couldn't tell for sure, because I'd thrown the other list away. My new doctor told me that I needed to exercise, not only for my back, but for my good health in general. Aerobic exercise, stretching, and moderate toning would work wonders for my physical conditioning.

With five years of maturing under my belt, I listened this time. I started an exercise program that I've never really quit. I did the back exercises for a few months, but with the regimen of aerobics and circuit training I was doing, I felt I didn't need additional back exercises.

I went on a practical regimen, going to a gym or athletic club four times a week. I'd put in a few miles on either a track or a treadmill, and then go through the weight circuit. After an hour, I'd work up a sweat. My wife went with me, working on her own program. I believe it's better to have a workout partner than to try exercising alone.

For the next twenty-four years, I had no major problems with my back. Yes, my right leg would hurt some on long drives, but nothing serious. However, five years ago, my wife and I began working out at a university aerobic center. I was physically fit and watching college-age students doing exercises on sophisticated equipment. I found at sixty-four years of age I could do those exercises as well as they could.

Beware—here enters the male ego. For all the years since my second back problem, I'd been using common sense while exercising. Now I had a vision of The Fountain of Youth. I increased my lap times on the track. I added weights to my circuit training. I added additional exercises, including back presses, abdominals, and inclined sit-ups. I felt great.

For three and a half years, I gained muscle, endurance, and energy. But the problem with men is we don't see our limitations. I kept adding another five-pound weight here and another set there. One day, I finished doing my workout, which included four sets of eight incline sit ups. I walked down the hill to my car and said to my wife, "Boy, my back hurts."

"You should see a doctor," she said. "Remember what happened before."

"Oh, this is nothing like that."

Two months later, I had to have an MRI, the pain was so bad. My doctor looked at the results and sent me to a neurosurgeon. We reviewed the tests together. "Well, Mister Wetterman, you've hurt your back before. You have old injuries to the L-1 and L-3 areas of your spine. But they are not the problem. This bulge here..."

I looked at the area where he pointed and could see the spot clearly.

"This area is the culprit. Right here between the L-4 and L-5 region of your spine."

I explained my regimen and told him I wanted to be right back working out as soon as I could.

"I want that for you, too," he said. "But let's go back to being sensible. You need to lower your weights. You need to stop the inclined sit-ups and maybe the abdominals and back presses. And that's only after this condition is back under control."

He referred me to a pain management clinic, and I had two injections into the area to reduce the swelling. For the third time, I followed the same directions given to me thirty-four years earlier. My pain level when I went to see the neurosurgeon was a twelve on a scale of ten. Now the pain is a three.

I don't like taking pain medication, but I do when necessary. I follow the orders of my doctors. Today, I'm still at the gym four times a week. I'm still on the track and doing weights. But the machismo has been brought under control out of necessity. I understand now about the balance between "use it or lose it" and "act your age."

I am about to turn seventy. I have advice for men like me who are working at aging in good grace and good health. Pace yourself. Know your physical and emotional limits. Think before you try something you're not either prepared or able to do. Be active. Follow your doctor's advice—and your wife's too.

Do I plan on being at the gym when I'm eighty? You bet I do. I'll be on the track, and I'll be working the weight circuit. But I'll be sensible and I won't try to act like I'm twenty-one.

~ Bill Wetterman ~

Back UP

I was surfing a big wave at the Banzai Pipeline in Hawaii when the whole thing collapsed on me. I was driven to the bottom, smashing my back on the sharp coral.

No, I was descending the Matterhorn after summiting. My climbing partner, who I was roped to, slipped and fell, leaving me to heroically haul him back up over the precipice, straining my back severely.

No, I was skydiving on my 500th jump when the primary chute and the back-up chute both failed and I fell over a thousand feet, my fall and back broken by the trees that saved my life.

Here's the less glamorous truth. I was cleaning the garage and decided to nudge a box of *National Geographic* magazines to the side, to give my wife some extra room to get her car in the garage. The pain was instant. Lower back. I hunched over, howling and swearing at myself.

I knew the box was heavy. I had needed help placing it where it was during our recent move into our dream house by the beach. That's why I'd opted to just give it a little nudge—and not try to lift it—the few inches to make the extra room for Marla's car.

And that had been enough to damage the facet joint and put me in what was to become permanent suspension of my forty-year surfing career, and pretty much everything else athletic.

First I tried just resting it to let it heal. I was very fit from surfing three to four times a week at my local world class surf spot, where fitness, like in basketball, is king. After a month and a half of disciplined abstinence, regular icing and personal Pilates instruction, I had to do something more physical or go crackers.

Golf seemed pretty benign at first. It had been a sport I'd long joked wasn't a real sport because it wasn't really athletic. I had said I might try it when I couldn't surf anymore, which I'd assumed would be a full decade later.

It turns out there is more athleticism to golf than I'd imagined, a lot of it very demanding on the lower back. After a month or so of doing "work arounds" with my fledgling golf swing, I had to lay off for fear of exacerbating my back injury that much more.

I sought out referrals to back doctors. All the non-surgical roads led to one practice, so that's where I went. A facet injection was advised, so that's what we did. And I was immediately cured. At least that's how it felt, for ten days.

I felt so certain of this I went out and bought a new tennis racket and tennis shirt and started hitting balls with my wife to get back into competitive form. For ten days.

Then the pain returned.

The next recommendation was an epidural. Yep, an epidural, the injection for pain they administer to women during childbirth.

No effect at all.

I was advised to work on my core at the gym.

I hired a trainer who recommended Somatics, so I did that for a month with no benefit.

Next I auditioned yoga studios. At the first place, the standing poses were too painful and demanding. At the second place, the room was so hot I couldn't breathe. The third was just right but it went out of business within the month and the owner and head yogini moved to Costa Rica.

Then came a sense of futility and a foray into depression as it became clear that my problem was incurable. I thought I was doomed to watch others from the sidelines—doing what I'd done with expertise and aplomb my entire life—ride sparkling pure ocean waves.

I had robbed myself of physical freedom, and I had constant moderate to strong pain, beginning upon awakening and not abating until I lay down at night. It was my constant companion and adversary.

Next came the pills to dull the pain but they didn't really work, at least not with unacceptable side effects, so they had to go. I was just going to have to devise a mental approach to "deal with it."

I resolved to just tough it out every day, to simply do the best I could one day at a time, and not become a complainer. So that's what I've done, for the past ten years.

Being crippled in this way got me out of a lot of yard work and fix-its around the house, but it was also humiliating to have to hire someone to do the work and to pay for things I used to do for free for myself. I became the talkative and probably overbearing supervisor to hired helpers, all tolerant to the last man. I'd been given a glimpse into old age, and it sucked.

Besides surfing I am also an artist and writer and I'd been meaning to write "my book" for decades. I'd spent a year at Cape Romanzof in the Arctic weather outpost my last year in the Air Force, a year deserving documentation, so I set out to do that.

I began painting again in earnest, growing brave enough to paint in public. My art grew from sketching and furtive pastels into full-fledged oil and watercolor paintings, my canvasses growing in size too, up to an oil triptych five feet high by twelve feet wide overall, my skills growing with each new work.

Not the same as surfing, or even golf, but a workout nonetheless.

I'm a voracious and curious reader by nature so all this "down time" provided me the opportunity to accelerate my reading schedule. Since the more demanding books demanded, duh, more of my attention and, consequently, less attention to the constant pain, I headed for the classics, historical and modern, discovering a thirsty penchant for philosophy, world history and current world events.

I also learned how to meditate to calm my mind. I started each day with prayer and meditation, a practice I continue to this day. It centers me and calms me, and I can do it any time during the day when I start getting frustrated and angry at my situation.

I had been a photographer since my teens, so I bought a four-by-five view camera and went old school, where discipline and fidelity to tradition are key to a more deliberate process than the quick affairs of the thirty-five millimeter format. This was Ansel Adams territory technically and I thrived on the challenge of making crisp well-metered negatives and the stunning large sharp exhibit prints they allow.

I stumbled into sculpture and worked for two years straight

pouring hot metal aluminum and bronzes of an expressive human figure I invented. I am encouraged to enter them in public art competitions for production into heroic pieces eight feet tall for display in urban environments.

I even took flying lessons because that is something I can do sitting down that allows me to move, literally. I love to move through time and distance and flying allows that.

A couple of months ago I went to my back pain management doctor, also a surfer, and he suggested it had been some time since we'd tried the facet injection treatment. Since timing is everything, he suggested we try it again. My insurance covered it so we did it, twice within a two-week period... and it took!

For two months now, my worst pain, what I've endured for over a decade, is gone.

My back is still sore as my muscles rediscover themselves gingerly—I'm not paddling out at Pipeline any day soon—but I'm getting better.

Without the pain my demeanor is better, lighter, brighter, and the jokes and banter come more easily again.

My book is finished and in search of a publisher. I have over twenty sculptures I'm putting patinas on and preparing to launch into the world. I have at least two paintings in the works at any given time.

And somewhere during all this a cartooning muse emerged in me and I now regularly submit my cartoons to *The New Yorker* for publication.

Reach for the stars, right, because you're liable to snag a planet? It's true.

The temptation is to say it's all the result of poor judgment, of a mistake I made trying to boost that box of *National Geographic* magazines, but I'm more inclined to call it fate.

Better yet, call it destiny.

I used to curse that year in the Arctic and my time in the military as wasted. Now I've gotten a book out of it. One that, if I do say so myself, has merit and style beyond what I might have expected of myself before I began it.

I body surf now instead of riding boards with the crowds. It's a more intimate connection with the sea and one I have grown to relish.

Much of what I have read this last decade had been on the "some day" list for years.

Now I own that knowledge.

I have learned that it is true that when one door closes another opens. You just have to stop focusing on the one that's closed and jiggle the knobs of the other ones until the right ones open.

And there are lots of doors.

~ James Daigh ~

A Long
and Bumpy
Road to Relief

I awoke one morning with a stiff neck from "sleeping funny." Over the next several weeks, the stiffness, bordering on pain, came and went. Then at times, I'd feel a sudden intense spasm when I turned my head or looked up or down. I used over-the-counter remedies without success, finally prompting me to make an appointment with my doctor. I hoped to nip my "pain in the neck" in the bud.

The doctor prescribed physical therapy three times a week for eight weeks, but the discomfort persisted. Eventually, he ordered X-rays, an MRI, and an ultrasound which revealed some arthritic changes and disc degeneration. The next step was referral to a pain management specialist.

After reviewing the test results and examining me, that doctor scheduled me for a cervical epidural steroid injection in the hospital while under anesthesia. It seemed a little early for such an extreme measure, but I was willing to try it. The procedure had no effect, however, so the doctor prescribed analgesic medication and outlined exercises to perform at home.

After no improvement, it was back to the hospital to try a

facet joint injection, again under anesthesia. Still no reprieve, so I continued with the medication and neck and back exercises.

I also began using a transcutaneous electrical nerve stimulation (TENS) unit attached to the skin by adhesive pads and wires. That helped manage the pain but only for as long as I used the TENS unit, no more than an hour at a time. On the next few visits, the doctor injected increasing amounts of steroids into my neck, but those improved neither my worsening condition nor my mood.

Then it was on to acupuncture... six weeks of needles, needles, and more needles. The only benefit I received came from the soothing upper-body massage preceding each acupuncture treatment. Now the pain traveled intermittently from my neck up into the back of my skull and around to my throat. I was beginning to lose my sunny disposition.

After all of these failed measures, the pain management specialist referred me to a neurologist. After examining me, the neurologist prescribed even stronger meds. On my next office visit, he administered a nerve block. More time passed with no improvement. So he ordered a brain MRI and an electroencephalogram (EEG) to rule out the possibility of brain tumor or stroke as the underlying cause.

Preparing for an EEG is a tug-o-war between your mind's wants and your body's needs. I was instructed to try to remain awake all night so that comparison could be made the following morning between wakeful and sleeping brainwave activity. Since the goal was to fall asleep during the testing, I had to find a good support system to help me stay awake the night before.

I have a friend who is a night owl and doesn't go to bed until at least 3:00 a.m. She said she'd call me before retiring for the night. Another friend is a runner who gets up around 5:00 a.m. for her morning jog. She agreed to call me as soon as she awoke. I have another friend who gets up frequently during the night to use the bathroom. She promised to call me every time she had to pee.

Earlier that evening, I'd worked my patrol shift as a volunteer with my local police department. Afterward, I wandered into dispatch to chat for a while before heading home. It was a fairly uneventful night, so they invited me to stay as long as I wished since I had to be up anyway. But I remembered the friends who said they'd call me periodically during the night. I decided to leave so they wouldn't worry when my phone went unanswered.

I got home about 3:30 a.m. and watched a little TV, straightened up the house, and played endless games of Solitaire on the computer until a beautiful sunrise greeted me. My appointment wasn't until 10:30 a.m. so I still had a lot of time to kill. Then the phone rang. It was the EEG technician asking if I could come in at 8:00 a.m. Oh, merciful Heavens, yes!

I drove the couple of miles to the facility where the technician got me settled comfortably in a recliner. She "glued" flat metal discs about the size of a nickel to strategic places on my scalp and lowered the room lights so I could drift off to blessed sleep. The sticky paste would wash out with a good shampooing afterward, she assured me. The electrodes were connected by wires to a machine that read my brainwaves to determine if the patterns were normal or abnormal. They could detect everything from stroke to brain tumor to epilepsy. I had none of these maladies. Good news, bad news. I was no closer to finding a solution to my neck pain.

I took matters into my own hands then and made an appointment with an orthopedic surgeon. I was able to see him within the week, armed with my bulging folder of medical data. He reviewed the information, examined me, and concluded that I had the aforementioned arthritic changes, bone spurs, and three herniated discs! The only viable solution at this point was a procedure called an anterior cervical discectomy and disc fusion. He'd remove the three offending discs (at levels C4, C5, and C6), and the bone spurs, through an incision made at the front of my neck. He would replace them with discs obtained from the bone bank, bracing them with a metal bracket and screws. The frontal incision would leave minimal scarring and less healing pain, he said.

I carefully weighed the pros and cons and then had the surgery, spending three days in the hospital. Once home, I ate only soft foods at first due to a sword swallower's sore throat, even cutting the painkillers in half in order to down them. I wore a cumbersome cervical collar for six weeks and an electronic bone fusion stimulator attached to my neck by adhesive pads for six months. They became my new best friends, along with physical therapy and massive doses of patience.

So after all of these efforts, was it worth it? The spinal

surgery was indeed the answer. I can turn my head once again, and I'm finally pain free. Hallelujah!

~ Annette Langer ~

Finally, Help Is on the Way!

Help for neck and back pain comes in many forms, and what works for one person may not work for another. Many of my patients tell me that they want to try whatever worked for their friend or family member. While that may seem like a good plan when you're in pain, the truth is that your pain is your own—and what works for someone else isn't necessarily the right thing to do to help you. It may be, but the critical part of helping anyone with neck or back pain is to know what the diagnosis is (or at least what the mostly likely possibilities include—the differential diagnosis list), and which treatments usually work for that particular condition.

Step Into My Office

Imagine that you are sitting in my office, and we're having a discussion about your back pain. The way that I usually explain treatment options to my patients is in three categories with conservative care being the first one, injections as the second, and surgery as the third. On a whiteboard I would lay out the following options.

Treatment Options #1— Conservative Management
Conventional care:
Avoiding exacerbating activities
Relative rest (not bed rest, usually)
Medications (over the counter or prescription)
Physical/Occupational therapy
Modalities (e.g., ultrasound, electrical stimulation)

Other treatments that are sometimes tried:
Osteopathy/Chiropractic adjustments
Massage
Acupuncture
Biofeedback
Mind-body strategies (e.g., progressive muscle relaxation)

Treatment Options #2— Injections
Spinal injections (e.g., epidural steroid injections)
Muscle injections (e.g., trigger point injections)

Treatment Options #3 — Surgery
This may be recommended immediately, only after
someone has tried other treatment options, or not at
all—it depends on the diagnosis, the severity of the
symptoms, and the surgeon's belief that he/she can fix
the problem with an operation.

Sometimes I recommend treatment stepwise, so that someone begins with therapies in the first category and then proceeds to the second category. If those don't work, I then suggest a surgical consultation. But, it doesn't always work that way. There are times when a patient needs to see the surgeon right away or injections make more sense than oral medications and physical therapy. There are many patients for whom surgery will never be an option, because they are too sick with other medical issues or their back problem can't be fixed by an operation or they simply wouldn't consider surgery no matter what (all medical treatment is recommended by doctors but it is up to patients to decide what they want to pursue—so physicians need to be respectful of their wishes when they say that they would not consider back surgery; of course, the doctors still need to explain all of the options, including surgery).

The stories in this chapter highlight a number of important points. In James's case, he tried facet injections more than once. James wrote that his doctor said sometimes timing really makes the difference. This is very true. There are many times when a patient has said to me that he tried a treatment several months or even years ago. Whether the treatment worked then or not, it can be helpful to try it again. Over time, things change and it may be that treatments you've tried in the past will work again (if they did before) or may work now (if they didn't work before).

Bill reports how he had back problems over many years that changed over time. He tried both conservative therapies and spinal injections and didn't resort to surgery. Annette's story explains how she tried both conservative therapies and injections before ultimately deciding that surgery was the "only viable solution."

Help may come in many forms. There are likely therapies that you haven't tried that might have the potential to help you. Sometimes what you've tried previously will work now. Other times, it's a combination of treatments that makes the difference. In some cases, the surgeon's mantra—"a chance to cut, a chance to cure"—holds true. Surgery can be the ultimate solution for some people. No matter what, seek out medical advice from physicians who are experts at treating neck and back pain. Educate yourself about treatment options that may help you. And, when in doubt, get a second (or third or fourth) opinion!

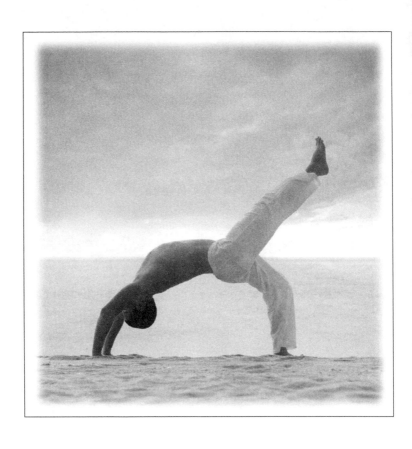

Chapter 7
Ahhh…
Sweet Relief

Pilates
Saved Me

I knew I was in trouble as soon as it happened. At sixty-four and halfway through a glorious vacation in New Zealand, I bent over to put clean clothes in my suitcase and then immediately straightened up as my back went into a spasm.

I cried out, "Oh no! Peter, I've pulled my back," hobbled to a sturdy chair, and sat down gingerly. "What should I do?"

My husband came across the room to me. "Where does it hurt?" he asked.

"My low back feels like I've been hit with a baseball bat," I replied.

He touched my back and I winced. "That makes it hurt more," I said.

"You should lie down on your side with your knees bent. Things may ease up if you are not moving. Let's see if an ice pack helps." He got ice and applied it to my back. Gradually the excruciating pain decreased... a bit.

By slowing down my schedule, I managed to see the sights. The unrelenting discomfort was a constant companion. I was determined to tough it out.

I said to my husband, "Can you please carry our suitcases? I can't lift anything without it hurting more."

The thirteen-hour flight home was miserable. Peter said, "You should walk as much as possible on the plane." I found there are limits to how much walking one can do on a 747. I ended up needing a wheelchair to meet me after our connecting flight from Los Angeles to Colorado the next morning.

We had been through similar issues with my husband's spine. Ten years ago, he developed leg pain with tingling in both feet and eventually had surgery.

I didn't want an operation unless absolutely necessary. I saw my primary care physician, did six weeks of physical therapy, used ibuprofen, and quit lifting anything that weighed more than a carton of milk. I wasn't much improved.

The physical therapist said, "We've done all we can."

The distress in my back and now down my leg was awful. I walked with a limp, constantly aware of the torment. I couldn't go hiking or biking. The pain pills didn't help; I was miserable. It was time to face reality.

We went to Denver to see Peter's neurosurgeon. I had my MRI in hand as my family practice physician said, "I'm afraid you're having the same problem Peter had ten years ago."

As Peter drove to my appointment, I said, "I'm dreading surgery. If there is any other option, I'll try it. An operation scares the heck out of me."

It seemed to take forever, but an hour and a half later Peter parked in front of the neurosurgeon's building. In minutes, I was being examined.

After going over my films and repeating some tests, the

doctor said, "Okay, I have good news and bad news. Which do you want to hear first?"

"Tell me the bad news. That way whatever the good news is will help cheer me up."

"You have two discs that are partially out. If this were six months down the line, I'd say it's time for surgery. The good news is, at this stage there's a 50% chance they'll go back in."

I thought out loud. "There is a new Pilates class in a physical therapy practice in Fort Collins. Do you think it would help?" I knew Pilates works on the deep muscles of the abdomen.

"Yes, it's known to strengthen the core muscles, which support the back. Avoid moves that aggravate the stabbing pain down your leg." Then he said, "I can refer you for a steroid shot to help with the pain."

His office manager scheduled that appointment in Fort Collins.

I was elated! Riding home, I told Peter, "I'll sign up for Pilates. I'm lean, but could lose a few pounds; I'm not sure if it will help, but it feels right. And I'll give up digging in my garden."

Four days after the steroid injection, my pain much improved, I went to the first class. The instructor was a slender woman, a physical therapist in her early thirties who really knew her stuff. Before things started, I introduced myself.

"Hi, Cindy, I'm here because of back problems. I'll need your help knowing if any of the moves might cause further injury."

Cindy listened sympathetically. "It sounds like you've got good motivation to take the class. I'll tell you which exercises you shouldn't do and give you some substitutes. Skip anything that causes you pain."

As we went through the Pilates moves, Cindy told me adaptations. "Don't even try the 'rolling like a ball' exercise; it squashes your vertebrae like a jelly donut and is exactly what you must not do. However, tightening your abs and balancing on your butt with your feet off the floor will strengthen your core muscles without hurting your back." Lo and behold, I could do that!

I liked the class. I lost ten pounds and transferred to the Pilates classes at the gym we belonged to. I enjoyed the new instructor and she incorporated the alternatives I had learned from Cindy. I attended sessions twice a week. Initially, my back symptoms didn't change much but I started to loosen up some of my muscles and always stopped doing anything that hurt.

It was a compatible group of Pilates regulars. Several were old friends. We began meeting in the gym's coffee shop after class; our camaraderie was a potent motivator.

After eighteen months of twice-weekly classes, I declared to the instructor, "Pilates has saved me from back surgery."

She nodded and said, "It takes about that long to begin to see results. I'm pleased you've made progress. Keep it up and you may never need that operation."

After four years, I'd had only one flare-up of back pain. I increased the classes to three times per week. Now it's been six years. My back has returned to normal.

I've done stretching and a few Pilates moves on the days

I'm not in class and incorporated breathing exercises for stress management.

I'm convinced that Pilates and a positive attitude saved me from back surgery. I'm committed to doing those exercises until I die... which, with my strong healthy body will likely be many years from now.

~ Lynnette C. Jung ~

Cat's Pose

W hen I was thirty, the only person I knew my age who had a back problem was a friend who had been in a bad boating accident. And she had a real back problem. She had suffered for years in pain. I had no idea how bad it was for her despite her phone calls and the days that she lay on her back unable to move. My health issue had always been migraines. If she wanted to talk pain, my head was where pain lived in my body.

One day when I was thirty-three I was toting around my young, but large, toddler on my hip and I bent down to pick up a toy. Suddenly pain shot through my back. Grasping my side, I put my daughter down and winced. I lowered myself slowly into a chair. And while she toddled off, I worried. How was I going to get through the rest of the day with a small child? What about the next day and the next week?

I knew my body was weak—especially my stomach and back. During pregnancy, and after the baby was born, I hadn't worked out like I had before I was pregnant. But I didn't have the energy, much less the time, to work out. I was so tired all the time.

As I sat there in pain, looking at my daughter, who had fortunately found something to play with, I realized—officially—that I was in terrible shape.

I called my mom, who is a nurse and is married to a man

who has had his share of back issues. Her suggestion was to take ibuprofen, try to rest (I rolled my eyes), and limit the time I spent picking up and holding my daughter (eye roll again). After a few days of consistent ibuprofen I was much improved. I went back into the nice cozy land of denial and went on my merry way.

A year later, I was pregnant with my second child and I started having back pain again—this time sciatica. I went into a tailspin again. I had actually gotten back in shape again before this pregnancy, but then I found that I simply couldn't muster any strength while pregnant and chasing my two-and-a-half-year-old around.

My desperation was increasing and the acetaminophen (no more ibuprofen) I could take was doing little to help ease my pain and discomfort.

I called my boating-accident friend and explained my back pain.

She told me to stretch, and suggested a few exercises.

"Yeah, right," I replied. "I'll just stretch and everything will be fine again."

Fortunately, she didn't hang up on me.

She walked me through the stretches. Most I recognized from yoga classes and general exercise classes. They seemed so wimpy and simple that I didn't really think they would work, but I was willing to give them a try.

For five to ten minutes a day, I went through a series of very simple stretches like lying on my back, legs straight and pulling one leg to my chest and holding it. Then I switched to the other leg. I also held both knees to my chest and rocked gently from side to side.

My all time favorite, and where I spent most of my time, was doing what they call in yoga the "cat's pose." On all fours, I would "tuck in" my enormous stomach, round my back, look down at the floor, and suck up my belly as far as I could. Then I would do the opposite, look up, push my belly toward the floor and arch my back. After a few times I could feel my back relax. Sometimes I would stay on all fours in a neutral position—I was just so glad not to be on my feet!

After a week, I couldn't believe how much better I felt and how simple the exercises were. I simply had to be disciplined enough to stay with it and do them. But they were so simple, and the repercussions of not doing them were so much worse, that I did them regularly.

Since then I have worked those exercises into my regular workout regime, pregnant or not, and so far, so good with the back pain. I have always been an animal lover, but now I have a whole new respect for the cat. Perhaps its healthy back is why it has nine lives.

— Jennifer Quasha —

Positioning Myself to Be Pain-Free

I ce packs, ibuprofen and massages had become a routine part of my existence. Every five to six weeks, I would wake up with a stiff neck, or I would turn the wrong way in the course of my day and end up with what felt like a knotted up shoulder blade. The pain would radiate down my back, up into my neck and lead to a splitting headache. The pain came and went in this pattern over a three-year period.

I learned to live with and manage these episodes, but the regularity with which they occurred became more frequent. The flare-ups exhausted me physically and mentally. I made myself go about my daily tasks, but the pain was distracting. I often couldn't devote my full attention to anything because of the ache.

One day, I found myself resting on the couch watching an afternoon talk show. The guest on this particular day was a back expert. They were discussing the most common causes of back pain and how it could be treated and/or managed. Needless to say, I listened intently. What I learned completely changed my life for the better. The expert talked about sleep positioning being a major contributor to back pain. I learned that my back and neck did not get the support they needed when I slept on my stomach or my side. I had been a tummy sleeper for as long as I could remember! The good news was that a change of sleep position could help. I was ready to give it a shot!

I began to force myself to sleep on my back. This was not easy for me. It took me several hours to fall asleep those first few nights. I also caught myself turning to the side and having to readjust myself. I had to train my body to sleep in this new position. The training would pay off, though. After a week, back sleeping became much easier, and over the course of a few months, I noticed something. I hadn't had to buy any ibuprofen! It was working. I hadn't experienced any back pain.

I'm now about six months into my new sleep routine, and so far I've only had one flare-up in my back. Not surprisingly, it was after a few nights of slipping back into tummy sleeping. I know that there are a number of reasons for back pain and that what has worked for me might not work for someone else, but going "back" to sleep has positioned me to be pain-free.

~ Kimberly M. Hutmacher ~

My Amazing Toe

My toe is possessed. At least that's what my family says. Sometimes the middle toe on my left foot points to the left, completely perpendicular to my foot, and tucks behind the fourth toe and the little pinky toe. You can't make your toe do this if you try! The only way I can straighten my toe is by grabbing it and forcing it back into position. It is always trying to move to the left, so it is permanently angled away from my big toe and my second toe, pushing the fourth and fifth toes out of position too. It looks like my left foot is making that Star Trek "V."

The first time I watched my toe do this I was so scared I called my neurosurgeon at 11 p.m. and asked if I should go to the emergency room. I thought that I was having a complete spinal breakdown!

Sometimes I also get electrical jolts in my left foot and in my middle toe, the same feeling you get if you accidentally touch the metal on a plug while plugging it into an electrical outlet. Sometimes my left foot will squeeze together into a cylindrical shape in a horrendous cramp. You can make this scrunched up shape with your hand but you can't do this with your foot, and I can't do it voluntarily—it just happens when it wants to.

My left calf goes through phases when it cramps so badly that I wake my husband in the middle of the night to rub it out. After a cramping incident I hobble around the next day until it calms down. I've learned to avoid pointing my left foot, as pointing can set off the cramp. I have to be careful inserting my left foot into a boot or skinny pants because I might point my toes by accident.

My back problems started ten years ago when I was in the best shape of my life, quite cocky, and lifted a heavy box improperly. An MRI showed a herniated disc, but after a year of proper exercises and care, as well as an extremely helpful steroid pack after all else failed, I was completely mended and had a relatively clean MRI. I hiked all over the place, including the demanding Inca Trail to Machu Picchu, skied, and did my normal activities, albeit carefully.

Then I was involved in what seemed like a minor car accident. I was hit from behind by a careless driver while I was stopped.

About a month after the accident I started having debilitating sciatic pain. I could barely walk and had to take a taxi to go one block in New York City. I was in pain 24 hours a day and could only sleep an hour at a time. When you are in that much pain you have to be very careful not to be grumpy so I over-compensated. I must have looked like I was on some kind of happy pill, the way I smiled at everyone and spoke so gently! I had to be particularly careful when I tried another steroid pack to see if that would help. Those can really change your behavior, making you loud and aggressive.

I ended up having an L4-L5 hemilaminectomy and the pain relief was immediate. All I took after the surgery was Tylenol, despite the lengthy procedure and the four-inch scar in my back.

If you have never had spinal surgery, you might be wondering what the recovery is like. For months, I couldn't bend forward to brush my teeth, couldn't shave my legs, and couldn't put on socks. But it was all worth it to end that pain and walk again.

It took a couple of years of diligent exercising to recover from the injury but I was finally back in business. Off we went to Chile to visit my son and his girlfriend during their semester abroad. On the first day of a four-day excursion to Easter Island, I dropped the soap in the shower, stepped on it, and flew through the air, landing smack on my back. My left leg went into a horrible cramping spasm from hip to toes. It was the worst pain I have ever felt, worse than childbirth, worse than anything I felt after the car accident.

It took an hour just to move me from the tub to the bed and I screamed for hours. The full-leg cramp never let up. There was no way I was going to see a doctor on tiny Easter Island. Luckily, Chile is one of those countries that allow the sale of mild narcotics over the counter, so I was able to dull the pain somewhat.

I could not put any weight on my left leg, but I was determined to see everything. We couldn't leave anyway. Easter Island is that island in the middle of the South Pacific with the mysterious 70-foot-tall carved heads. It is 2,300 miles from Chile and 2,200 miles from Tahiti. There were only four airline flights per week—two to Chile and two to Tahiti, so I was stuck there for a couple of days whether I liked it or not. I hopped around the island on my right leg for the next three days with my husband or my son acting as a human crutch on my left side.

Upon my return to the United States, the neurosurgeon was mystified by my MRI. It showed a large cloud over the L4-L5 area. My doctor said he had never seen anything like it and he would have feared that it was a tumor except for the fact that it was the site of my previous surgery and my new injury. I still couldn't put any weight on my left leg so I sidled along walls and used furniture to support me as I limped around for the next month. I had very little sensation in the skin on top of my left foot and the back of my left calf. Try shaving your leg when you can't actually feel your skin! The doctor said that I had suffered serious nerve damage from the bathtub fall and that it could take up to two years for the nerves to recover. Over time, I regained the use of my left leg and I didn't even recognize my spine in the MRI I had six months later. The mysterious cloud had disappeared and when I looked at my MRI with my doctor, my L4-L5 area was the "cleanest" I had ever seen it, with virtually no herniation.

More than three years have passed. I have my "possessed" toe that moves by itself and my weird electrical shocks and my intermittent cramping. My left leg is much less flexible than my right leg, but I hike, ski, and do almost everything that I want to do. I continue to do the exercises the doctor gave me after my surgery and I think I am still improving. I am very careful about lifting things—I only fill grocery bags half full, I make three trips down the stairs to carry a load of laundry, I ask strangers for help—and I don't do certain things that might stress my back such as horseback riding or amusement park rides. I do not point my toes! This is how I live my life and it is fine. I figure we all have something wrong with us by the time we are in our mid-fifties and I am thankful every day that this is my thing, since it could be a lot worse!

— Amy Newmark —

Ahhh…
Sweet Relief

Healing your back takes time and patience. Many people with back pain will have nearly complete relief of their symptoms within two weeks. But, too often, the pain lasts much longer and is truly debilitating. One of the things that I spend a lot of time discussing with my patients is how in the old days doctors carried around black bags with their tools. I ask my patients, "If you had a black bag to control your pain, what would be the tools that are in the bag?" The idea of helping patients to develop their own "black bag" is really a metaphor for assisting them in identifying what tools they may be able to use at home if they have pain.

Many of my patients tell me that the worst part of having pain is not knowing how bad it will get and not having a way to control it. This worry is really fear about pain. In fact, there are a number of very interesting studies that have been done looking at how the fear of pain is often more disabling than the pain itself. So, as a medical doctor who treats a lot of people with back pain, I recognize that I need to treat not only pain but also fear.

This brings me back to my point about developing your own "black bag." Having a black bag doesn't mean that you don't need to check in with your doctor. I always recommend that people get excellent medical advice, and in fact, your physician can contribute some tools to your bag. The goal is to try and not have "emergency" situations in which you are in severe pain and unable to control it. Having a black bag will not prevent every emergency situation, but it will help to prevent some of them and it will also help to reduce worry and fear about having uncontrolled pain.

Finding the Right Tools for Your Black Bag

I know from having many conversations with patients that it's not always obvious which tools should go into your black bag. So, I start by asking them this general question: What tools do you have at home that may help you to control your pain? If they aren't sure, then I ask them a series of questions about what has helped them in the past. Anything that helps, even a little bit, is something to consider putting in the bag.

Add a hot pack or cold pack. Moist heat, such as a hot bath or shower can also work well. Use either heat or cold or both — depending on your own experience with how these make you feel. Be careful, though, because both heat and cold can cause burns if they are used for too long or at too extreme a temperature.

Move your body. Safe movement is usually helpful to manage pain. Tools may include stretching exercises, yoga, Pilates, swimming or any other form of exercise (if it helps). Rest may also be a tool. However, it's important to know that strict bed rest usually makes you feel worse, not better. Plus, it's not good for the rest of your body. So, when it comes to rest, usually what doctors recommend is avoiding activities that make the pain worse, rather than going to bed and staying there for days or weeks.

Find a comfortable position during the day. Another component of avoiding exacerbating activities includes assessing what you do every day and how you might be able to get your body in a better position. For example, if you have neck pain, using the speakerphone or an earset is very helpful. If you have low back pain, a supportive chair at work and lumbar support cushion in your car is a good idea.

Find a comfortable position at night. Mattresses and pillows may make things better (or worse). The only way to know if a certain mattress or pillow will help you is to try it out. Back belts and neck braces are usually not a good idea to use as they promote stiffness and weaken the muscles that support the spine.

Lighten your load. This can mean lifting less weight (lighten your laundry basket, buy a half gallon of milk instead of a full gallon, and so on). Or, it can mean losing weight (if you are overweight). Two things that help support your "core" (your core is the middle of your body—where most neck and back pain originates) include:

1) lessening the work that the core muscles have to do to support your body by lifting less and/or losing weight; and

2) strengthening your core muscles so that they can better withstand whatever stress they need to tolerate.

Tap into your mind-body connection. Mind-body tools for your black bag may include relaxation techniques, conscious and controlled breathing, meditation, imagery, hypnosis and biofeedback.

Talk to your doctor. Your physician may recommend some tools for your bag, too. Of course, I'm talking about things that people have access to at home, so surgery or injections wouldn't be tools for the bag, but over-the-counter and prescription medications count. You might find a TENS (transcutaneous electrical nerve stimulation) device helpful. TENS units may be used at home and are usually prescribed by doctors and physical therapists.

Take a minute to think about your own tools—you can even write down a list if you are so inclined. Sometimes it's helpful to see on paper what interventions you actually have on hand to control your pain. Thinking about your black bag can be quite enlightening and also empowering.

Should you use heat or cold to relieve your pain?

The answer to this is — it depends. But, there are some general guidelines. First off, it helps to know what high or low temperatures do to your body. Heat acts as a muscle relaxant, so if your pain is due to muscles that are in spasm, warmth usually helps. Cold does two things — it decreases inflammation and provides an anesthetic effect (by numbing the area). So, if inflammation is a problem, then a cold pack may help. Also, it might just feel good because of the anesthetic effect. Try them both and decide which one works best for you. For the back and neck areas, it's fairly safe to use heat as long as it's not too hot (and causes a burn). Ice packs are fine to use for about 20 minutes, but should be taken off after that time and then reapplied several hours later if needed.

Tools that Might Be in Your Black Bag

Medications
TENS unit
Comfortable pillow/mattress
Supportive chair for home/work/car
Hot pack/cold pack
Hot shower/bath
Exercises
Yoga/Pilates/tai chi
Diet
Lifting less weight
Mind-body strategies

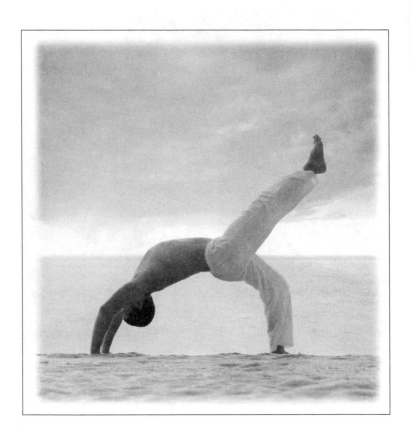

Chapter 8
Brush and Floss Your Back

Backed into
a Corner

"Come on, Evan, it's time to go," I said, as sternly as I could. It was late afternoon and my son and I were at the park. It was time to go home. But Evan wasn't budging. He plunked down on the grass and began wailing.

I didn't know what to do. I wanted to pick him up and haul him off to the car. But my back was killing me. Evan was thirty pounds of solid, squirming three-year-old.

I'd had a bad back for a long time, but my son usually was so obedient that this situation hadn't come up before. I couldn't think of a good solution. I blurted out the only thing that came to mind—and I didn't like it.

"Evan, if you don't come with me right now, I'll have to spank you," I warned.

Please, please get up, I pleaded silently. I'd never spanked my child and I didn't want to start now.

But he didn't get up. He just kept crying.

Reluctantly, I leaned down—yow, that hurt!—and pulled Evan to his feet. I tried to swat him on the behind, but had trouble finding it with him wriggling to break free. I tapped at him awkwardly. I'm not even sure I made contact.

Thankfully, it was enough. He came along with me to the car, still crying, but no longer balking.

That afternoon in the park convinced me that I had to do something about my back. I had let it go on far too long.

It all began after childbirth. In pregnancy, the body's ligaments loosen and stretch to accommodate the growing baby and coming birth. Afterward, they may not support a woman's joints and bones the way they once did.

I first noticed how severe my troubles were when we signed Evan up for swim lessons. He was still a baby, so it was a "mommy and me" class. We were in the pool with our babies, hoisting them in and out of the water, swishing them back and forth. Except after the first class it was clear this was going to be a "daddy and me" activity.

Over the next few years, my pain grew worse. I tried to compensate. I wore loose clothes. I got one of those grabber gadgets, so I didn't have to bend down to pick up toys. I slept on the floor.

Then one day, in one of those quick sideways motions you make without thinking, I reached down to pick up the cat and—OUCH! I felt a stabbing pain in my lower back.

This was pain of a different order. It radiated down into my left leg and immobilized me. I searched the Internet for solutions—moms are too busy to go to the doctor! I read that most back pains resolve themselves in six to eight weeks. Stupidly, I set that mental deadline.

Eight painful weeks dragged by, including the day of the

park tantrum. After that, I lost faith in the Internet and went to my doctor, who packed me off to physical therapy.

My therapist did what therapists do. At first, it was just gentle manipulation of my legs, up and down, back and forth. Soon, she brought in a TENS unit—an electrical gadget that stimulates and relaxes the muscles that have tightened around the strained area.

Despite the treatment, I was dismayed to find that my pain worsened over the next few weeks. I cried to the therapist that I wanted to stop.

"Have patience," she said. "It feels worse for a while, and then suddenly, it gets better."

And she was right. Especially after she introduced me to what I fondly call The Rack. It's really not a medieval torture device, but a two-part cushioned traction table. At regular intervals, the parts separate and then close back together. The outward motion stretches out the vertebrae, relieving your pain for a few blissful moments.

I loved my rack! It was in a private room. I'd take a book in with me and read uninterrupted for a blessed half hour while the table whirred quietly out and back.

Eventually, I had to do the hard work. In the exercise area, I was given a routine meant to strengthen my muscles, especially the abdominal ones that support the back. I used resistance bands and gently worked my arms and legs on the machines.

A few weeks later, I was thrilled to graduate. I could accomplish daily tasks again, and I was smarter about it. I bent my knees to lift things. I got up and moved around after sitting for a while. I bought a firmer mattress. I did my floor exercises.

After a few years, though, the pain began to assert itself again. I was carrying around those extra pounds you tend to accumulate in mid-life. My blood pressure was high, and my doctor was suggesting medication.

Thankfully, I figured out how to help myself. I joined a gym and began to swim laps three times a week. In the water, your back troubles virtually disappear. I gradually worked my way up from ten minutes to half an hour. Afterward, I'd sit in the hot tub and let the jets massage my back.

It's been seven years now, and I still swim every few days. It keeps my back pain at bay, and I've lost thirty pounds to boot. The other day, I picked up three ten-pound bags of flour, curious to see how heavy those extra pounds feel, whether you happen to be wearing them or hoisting them.

Those thirty pounds of flour reminded me of that day in the park when I was forced into a decision. I never again had to try to spank my son. Today, at age twelve, he is an easygoing and agreeable young person, and I'm thankful for that—because even with a good back, I don't think I could lift nine bags of flour!

— Nancy B. Kennedy —

Hooray for Heated Seats!

My back starting acting up about the same time my car did. They were both old and worn out. Thankfully, my doctor found no serious problems with my muscles or spine. "You're no spring chicken, you know," she said. "The older we get, the more our backs tend to hurt. Back pain is the second most common neurological problem in the country, right behind headaches. The best advice I can give you is to keep moving. Take an anti-inflammatory when you're really uncomfortable. And direct heat helps."

My mechanic's advice was a lot more blunt. "Sell that heap of junk," he said, "before you have to pay to have it hauled away."

So I did. And I bought a low-mileage used car without a lot of bells and whistles. No satellite radio. No navigation system. No moon roof. But there was one luxury I insisted upon—heated front seats. I flipped the driver's seat switch to high as I pulled out of the dealership parking lot. Within seconds, the backs of my leg grew warm. So did my tush. Best of all was the heat that radiated across my lower back.

I stopped for groceries on the way home and, not wanting any dents or dings on my new set of wheels, parked at the far end of the parking lot. A brisk walk into the store, a brisk cruise through the milk and bread aisles, a brisk walk back across the parking lot and I was done.

Without a twinge of back pain.

I used the seat heat when I drove my daughter to piano lessons that afternoon. But instead of sitting in the car thumbing through a magazine like I usually did during the half-hour wait, I strolled around the block. My back didn't bother me at all.

In the weeks that followed the purchase of my car, I fell into a routine. A few minutes of radiating heat any time I needed to drive somewhere, followed by a few minutes of walking. I found myself taking less and less pain medicine. My walks grew longer and brisker. As a chilly spring became a not-so-chilly summer, I wondered whether the heated car seat would be too uncomfortable. No worries. I simply used the "low" setting on the seat warmer and bumped the air conditioning up a notch.

And I kept on walking.

Is my back pain gone for good? No. Every now and then, I feel that familiar pang that reminds me that I'm no spring chicken. But I know what to do about it. I take a quick drive. Then I take a long walk.

And I remain forever grateful that I was able to find a good used car with no bells and whistles. Except for the very one my poor, aching old back needed.

~ Jennie Ivey ~

A Mom's
Back Pain Plight

Since having children, I had severe back pain. Doctors told me it was probably from lifting babies and toddlers and carrying them around on one hip. I knew it initially stemmed from an old water-skiing accident, but lifting and carrying young children certainly exacerbated the problem. I had seen many doctors, been prescribed heavy-duty meds, and been in and out of physical therapy. What was worse is that I was told it was a chronic condition and I would have to learn to live with the back pain.

I finally found a doctor who specialized in lower back pain and seemed to understand my plight, not just as a back pain sufferer, but also as a mommy. While looking over my MRI, she paused for a moment and made a funny noise, almost like a woodpecker pecking at an old tree. Then she turned to me and said, "You have the spine of an eighty-year-old woman."

"But I'm only thirty!" I screeched. "What does that mean?"

She pointed to the lower vertebrae on my MRI. "These are vertebrae L5, L4 and even L3. See how thin they are compared to your other vertebrae?"

I nodded.

"They should be thicker and spongy, but yours look worn down, like an old lady's spine. Probably from a previous injury."

My mind raced back to the water skiing incident when I was a teenager. "So what will I be like when I'm eighty?" I asked, sort of joking but not really. Visions of walkers and wheelchairs now flashed in my head.

"You will probably need surgery at some point, to fuse the vertebrae. That often helps."

The doctor continued to examine me. My back was out of line as well and one hip was higher than the other. "Often carrying children around on one side and lifting children can cause back pain," she said.

I nodded again. I could see that being a problem. I had been lifting babies for three years now.

"You could also lose some weight. Excess weight means more pressure on your body, your feet and of course, your spine."

I nodded again. I knew that was a problem. After my second child, getting the baby weight off was hard, if not impossible. I had little time to take care of my family, let alone take care of me. I let out a long, deep sigh.

"I'll send you to a physical therapist and in the meantime, exercise at home, take this prescription, use ice packs and by all means, stop carrying your kids around!" She smiled, knowing that often it was hard to refuse a two-year-old who wanted nothing more than to be picked up by Mommy. I scoffed at the medicine she prescribed and waved the prescription in the air. "These make me so tired," I said. "I can't function as a mom!"

"I know—take them at night when you'll be asleep anyway. They will help."

I followed the regimen as well as I could and my back soon got better. I was careful about bending over and picking things up, especially little ones. I let my husband Jeff help out more and encouraged nightly back rubs. He also helped me with my exercises.

Things were going well until the kids, my husband and I scrambled into my brother's pick-up truck for a fun outing at the beach. We were on vacation and Jon had a beach pass. The only problem was that we had to four-wheel-drive on a rocky road to get to the beach. We bounced and rocked and were jostled about to the beach and then four hours later, back. About halfway home I felt a dull ache in my lower back but ignored it. When we got home, hot and sandy and sunburned, and I slid out of the pick-up truck, an excruciating pain shot through my back and down my leg. It was so painful I let out a cry and fell to the ground. My brother and husband rushed over and picked me up but I could not stand on my own.

The muscles spasms in my back felt like a knife was continually being plunged in and out. My brother and Jeff carried me into the house and lay me down on my bed. Jeff sort of knew the drill, even though I had never had back pain this bad. He got me the ibuprofen, ice and started to massage my lower back while Jon watched the kids.

The next morning I could not get up. I could hardly move. I lay in bed and listened while I heard the laughter and conversation of my family enjoying their vacation. My children visited me throughout the day, showing me things they collected on the beach, kissing me with peanut butter and jelly-smeared faces and even sitting on the bed pretending to read me a story. Jeff continued to give me back rubs, helped me with the exercises my physical therapist suggested, cooked, cleaned, entertained, and played the role of both mom and dad. I hated it! I hated being catered to. I was not an invalid! I wanted to live life, not just watch it pass me by and although I rather liked not cooking or cleaning, I would have given anything to be able to do those things.

"You really need to get up and try to walk around," Jeff said. "Remember, moving is good, not bad."

Despite how much it hurt, I got up every few hours and shuffled around the room. After three days, my back was better and although it ached continually, the sharp pains subsided. I could walk and sit for short periods. I was sort of back in vacation mode, but severely restricted in what I could do.

When I got home, I resumed physical therapy and I resumed life, but from a different perspective. I realized that I could play an active role in my family's life, but I just could not do things I might have taken for granted before. Now, I never lift, push or pull heavy objects. I always ask for help. I don't ride horses, roller coasters that jerk the body suddenly or go four-wheeling. I don't rake leaves or shovel snow. I avoid any motion that might cause my back to go out or be strained. I buy shoes that support my feet, remember to have good posture and try to walk a lot. Moving, including swimming, has helped to strengthen my back and I've lost some weight too.

Sometimes there is a lot to remember and sometimes I strain my back. When it happens, I grab the ice, the ibuprofen and my husband. I take care of the problem before it does me in. I've realized that in order for me to take care of others, I need to take care of myself first. I'm not sacrificing anything either. It was hard at first to realize I just couldn't do things I always loved, like ride horses, but that was a sacrifice I was willing to make.

I'm sure I'll always have chronic back issues and that my spine is still like that of an elderly woman, but I've been back-pain-free for almost ten years. I've not seen a physical therapist in that time and the strongest medication I've needed is ibuprofen. I probably won't bungee jump like my seventy-year-old father-in-law, but I have no doubt I will be enjoying life.

~ Jennifer Bond Reed ~

May I Suggest?

Every time I see a moving truck go by two things happen to me. First, I get nervous, and second, my back starts aching. It has been my lot in life to have moved twenty-five times in forty years. I have seen too many moving boxes. I have packed and unpacked and lifted too many moving boxes. Not to mention things too big for boxes, like desks and dressers and tables and chairs. Were it not for developing a personal strategy for handling moves, I am certain I would be living with debilitating back pain by now.

In the process of helping friends with their moves, I have used these principles repeatedly and have always been surprised at how many of my tips have not occurred to them. I share them here in the hopes they will spare the reader's back as well.

One: SMALL BOXES. Always use small boxes for heavy items. Sounds logical but every time I did not pack for myself I invariably found the movers had plunked a heavy tool-box or power saw in the bottom of a huge box of canvas lawn chairs or such. Small boxes are easier to store, to stack, to lift, to transfer, and they put much less strain on your back. You can pick up a small box and still see the path at your feet. Large boxes can cause you to go blindly, thus risking a fall from tripping over an unseen item on your path.

Two: MULTIPLE TRIPS. A natural consequence of using

smaller boxes. It is much easier on your back to make two trips with a twenty-five pound box than strain for those fifty-pounders.

Three: DOLLIES/HAND-TRUCKS. Whatever you call those contraptions with two wheels and a ledge at the bottom and a sturdy steel frame and top handle, use them. Again, several small boxes can be easily stacked on these dollies, making transfer much easier. In fact, anything with wheels is useful. I have transferred heavy items in wheelchairs, play wagons, garden carts and office chairs with sturdy casters.

Four: TAKE THINGS APART. People are always amazed at how much furniture I can move by myself without hurting a muscle. One secret is taking apart anything that comes apart. I cannot grab a big dresser the way two hunky men can, but I have moved multiple pieces after removing the heavy drawers and doors. I had offered a huge desk to a church organization recently. Two men came to look at it and were mumbling about how to get it through the door. When they returned the next day with their truck I had the desk ready for them by the garage door. It had come from the factory in a box. What goes together in pieces comes apart in pieces! I never hurt a finger, let alone my back. (It came in forty-eight pieces. I broke it down to six.)

Five: SLIDERS. Right in there with wheeled dollies is using those wonderful sliders under furniture legs. I used an assortment of old plastic lids and coasters but now they have specially made items in assorted sizes. You can move an amazing amount of stuff across a room by giving it a shove on its sliders. Mats work as well on hardwood floors.

Six: STAGES/STEPS. I have discovered I can easily lift weight from waist level down to the floor using leg muscles but it is more difficult for me to get things from floor level up to shoulder level. So I use multi-level techniques. For example, I might lift a large printer from the floor to a low ottoman on wheels. Then I roll it over to the high desk it goes on and lift it from ottoman to desk. These halfway steps enable me to use arm or leg muscles as needed and allow me time to reposition rather than straining my back in a complicated sustained lift.

Seven: DIVIDE & CONQUER. I use the steps principle also to divide and conquer large loads. I learned this from my mother, who was boasting one day about the good deal she found on fifty pounds of potatoes. Mother loved potatoes and had her winter supply in her basement cold room. But I wondered how the little eighty-four-year-old had managed that. "Who put them in for you?" I asked. "I did it myself!" she proudly announced. Then she explained. The grocer had put them in the trunk of her car. When she got home she opened the sack and took out small pails. She filled each pail with about ten pounds and carried them into the house, little by little. Whether it's potatoes, birdseed or cases of canned goods, instead of putting your back out, divide the load into manageable portions.

Eight: ASK FOR HELP. There will be times when none of the above tips will be practical. You can remove a headboard and a footboard but you still have a queen-size box spring and mattress you cannot divide. There's always the fridge and stove and washer and dryer. Enlist help when you need it. With moving especially, one needs physical help, but you will find that the right help also brings psychological support. Sometimes our backs can be bent under emotional burdens as well as physical ones. In the past I have had friends come and clean my fridge for me when I was exhausted from packing. It's not that I wasn't able to clean my own fridge. It was the act of kindness. The chatting and humor we shared, the emotional support given that truly lifted the weight and suddenly made me feel less tired, less achy. Enlist help when you need it. Accept offered help if it is from someone you trust and with whom you are comfortable.

Nine: KNOW WHEN TO REST. Lastly, know when to rest. Among my friends and acquaintances, I have found most are driven to perform to high standards day in and day out. I see young mothers worn to a frazzle in caring for their families. I see men pushing themselves day after day to be good breadwinners. I see women juggling careers and families and doing a wonderful job of both. I see older people who could be sitting in rocking chairs choosing instead to be out there in the community keeping things going.

But we all have our limits and knowing our limits is vitally important. Whether it's after the movers have rolled up their quilted pads and closed the door of the truck and finally pulled away, or just Friday night after a long week—know when to quit. Know when enough is enough. When you need to pour that cup of tea and head for the recliner chair, or pull the blinds and crash on the bed. When we are over-tired we are more prone to mistakes, poor judgment, accidents or falls. Fatigue makes us tense and our backs feel it too. Take a deep breath. Relax. Your back will thank you.

— Phyllis McKinley —

Brush and Floss
Your Back

Taking care of your back is a lot like caring for your teeth. Daily habits, like brushing and flossing, make all the difference. While brushing and flossing won't guarantee that you'll never get a cavity, there's no doubt that these habits help prevent problems. My patients often tell me that they want me to fix their backs so that they never hurt again. I say, "That's a lot like going to the dentist and saying that you never want to have another cavity. It's just not possible."

However, what is possible is to "brush and floss" your back, so that you have fewer future problems and when they do occur, they aren't as severe. Backs are a lot like teeth — taking care of them pays off but doesn't prevent every problem.

So, here are some "brushing and flossing" tips for your back:

1. Strengthen your core. Try this simple test that I ask patients to do in my office. I have patients lie on their backs, fold their arms across their chests and then sit up without using their arms at all. When you do this, be careful not to straighten your arms or use them in any way to help you sit up. This is a simple test for "core strength." Many people have strong arms and legs but weak abdominal muscles (these help support

the back). If you can't easily do this, chances are you have a weak core, and need to do some strengthening exercises (to start you can try pelvic tilts and curl-ups—for further advice about how to do these, ask your doctor, physical therapist or a "trainer").

If your core is already strong, keep it strong by exercising it—for the rest of your life. Focus on your posture. Slouching is hard on your back, but we all tend to do it during the day. I always ask my patients if they are sitting in supportive chairs with good lumbar supports. Positioning your low back and neck to improve posture and support can relieve a lot of pain.

2. Stand up. Sitting for too long is hard on your back, so spend a good part of your day standing. Better yet, move around. Walk and stretch. Get your muscles contracting and your blood pumping.

3. Sit down. Are you confused? Well, here's the thing—our bodies are not made to stay in one position—either sitting or standing. So moving around and alternating between sitting and standing is the best thing for your back. The more you move, the better your back feels (and the rest of your body). Of course, some positions or activities will bother sensitive backs, so always do what feels good for your body.

4. Invest in good shoes. By "good shoes," I mean ones that are supportive and cushion your steps as you walk. The best ones are usually excellent running sneakers. The worst ones — high heels. Keep in mind that healthy, active people should be taking 10,000 steps a day. This means that every year your feet are taking close to 4 million steps. Every step counts and translates forces up your leg to your hip and back. Millions of forces that are just a tad more than they need to be add up to "back pain." So, invest in good shoes.

5. Throw your "good shoes" out. I know this is counterintuitive, but even when your investment still looks nice on the top, it's probably not working that well on the bottom (where you need it). The heels and soles of shoes often wear out long before the rest of the shoe does. Which means that your shoes may look good, but don't feel good to your back. I tell my patients to consider getting a new pair of shoes every six months or so — after 1-2 million steps. Of course this depends on how active you are, how heavy you are, how often you wear a particular pair of shoes, etc. The point here is — don't judge your shoes by how they look but by how they are cushioning every single step.

6. Relax! Relaxation techniques can help lessen pain by decreasing muscle spasm and focusing on pleasant or peaceful thoughts.

These are all fairly simple strategies which can become regular habits. Once they become part of your regular routine, like brushing and flossing your teeth, you won't even have to think much about them. Developing routines to care for your back usually leads to less pain and better function. So, brush and floss your back regularly!

Curl-up*

Exercises the central abdominal muscles

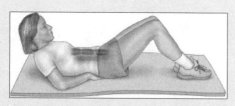

Lie on your back on a mat. Put your hands beneath the small of your back and bend both knees to help stabilize your spine. Slowly raise your head and shoulders just a few inches off the floor. Pause. Slowly lower your head and shoulders. Aim for eight to 12 repetitions. Rest and repeat the set.

*If you have osteoporosis, talk to your doctor before trying this exercise. He or she may recommend that you avoid it.

Reprinted with permission from the Harvard Health Publications Special Health Report: Strength and Power Training (2010)

Back strengthening exercises

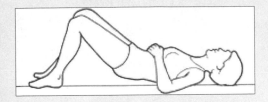

1. Lie on the floor on your back. Bend your knees and keep your feet flat on the floor. Squeeze your buttocks and pull your abdomen in toward your back. Your lower back should be pressed flat on the floor. Now raise your buttocks about an inch off the floor. Your lower back will lift slightly off the floor while your upper back remains flat. Hold for a few seconds before relaxing. Repeat 10 times.

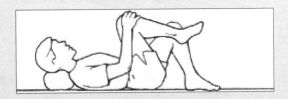

2. While lying on the floor on your back, with your head and neck supported, grasp your leg just below your knee. Pull your leg gently toward your chest. Hold for 20 seconds. Repeat on other side. Repeat 10 times.

Back strengthening exercises (continued)

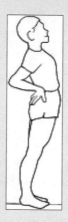

3. Stand with your feet slightly apart and your hands on the top of your buttocks. While looking up, push your hips forward slightly and gently bend backwards. Keep your knees straight. Hold for 10 seconds. Relax. Repeat 10 times.

Reprinted with permission from the Harvard Health Publications Special Health Report: Low Back Pain (2010)

If you brush and floss your teeth and back — every single day — there is no doubt that they'll be healthier!

Which technique is right for you?

By regularly practicing techniques that elicit the relaxation response, you create a well of calm to dip into as the need arises. As this chart details, these techniques can be especially beneficial under certain circumstances, but may not be suitable under others.

Method	What is it?	Especially beneficial	May not be suitable
Breath focus	Focusing on slow, deep breathing and gently disengaging the mind from distracting thoughts and sensations	If you have an eating disorder or tend to hold in your stomach; may help you focus on your body in healthier ways	If you have health problems that make breathing difficult, such as respiratory ailments, heart failure, or panic attacks
Body scan	Focusing on one part of the body or group of muscles at a time and mentally releasing any physical tension you feel there	For increasing your awareness of the mind-body connection	If you have had a recent surgery that affects body image or other difficulties with body image
Guided imagery	Using pleasing mental images to help you relax and focus	When you want to reinforce a positive vision of yourself or a goal you wish to reach	If you have intrusive thoughts that make imagery difficult; if you have difficulty with visualizations
Mindfulness meditation	Breathing deeply while staying in the moment by deliberately focusing on thoughts and sensations that arise during the meditation session	If racing thoughts make other forms of meditation difficult	If you find it too hard to commit the needed time
Yoga, tai chi, and qi gong	Three ancient arts that combine rhythmic breathing with a series of postures or flowing movements	At times when your mind is racing; whenever you find it especially hard to settle down and focus; if you wish to enhance flexibility and balance	If you are not normally active or have health problems or a painful or disabling condition; if so, speak with your doctor before starting any program of exercise
Repetitive prayer	Using a short prayer or phrase from a prayer to help enhance breath focus	If religion or spirituality is meaningful to you	If you are not religious

Meet Our Contributors

Mita Banerjee enjoys being a writer, teacher, mother, wife and friend. She is passionate about saving the environment, and spends much of her time encouraging that enthusiasm in the children of her neighborhood. She lives by the simple motto of doing (at least) one good deed a day. E-mail her at mitabaner@gmail.com.

Carisa Janelle (Wyrwas) Burrows, a Penn State graduate, hails from Johnstown, PA, and now lives in Pittsburgh with her loving husband Ralph. She began writing two years ago as a way of coping with several unexpected spinal surgeries and thanks her family for their unending support and love. E-mail her at carisaw@hotmail.com.

Now that **Emily Chase** has given up playing volleyball, she has more time for writing and speaking. Her seven published books include *Help! My Family's Messed Up* (Kregel, 2008) and her newest book, *Standing Tall After Falling Short* (WingSpread, 2012). Visit her at emilychase.com to learn more!

Brenda Cook is a veteran teacher with thirty-two years of classroom teaching experience. She enjoys reading, writing, traveling, and spending time with family and friends. Brenda is also actively involved in women's ministry at her church and participates in various mission opportunities.

James Daigh lives in Carlsbad, CA with his astonishing wife of thirty years, the mellifluous Marla. He is a poet, artist, magazine publisher and editor, filmmaker, photographer and cartoonist. His loves are poetry, drawing and painting, reading, acoustic guitar and travel.

Linda C. Defew calls rheumatoid arthritis a blessing in disguise. When it forced her to put needlework aside, her dream of writing took its place. Now, living on a farm with her husband and six dogs, she is thankful to God for a wonderful life. E-mail her at oldwest@tds.nct.

Terri Elders, LCSW, lives near Colville, WA, with two dogs and three cats. Her stories have appeared in multiple editions of the *Chicken Soup for the Soul* series. She's a public member of the Washington State Medical Quality Assurance Commission. E-mail her at telders@hotmail.com and read her blog at http://atouchoftarragon.blogspot.com.

Shawnelle Eliasen and her husband Lonny raise their five sons in Illinois. She home teaches her youngest children and writes about their adventures. Her stories have appeared in *Guideposts*, *MomSense*, *A Cup of Comfort* books, *Christmas Miracles*, *Christmas Spirit*, and several *Chicken Soup for the Soul* books. She blogs at Shawnellewrites.blogspot.com.

An ordained Baptist minister, **Malinda Dunlap Fillingim's** heart is full of precious memories of her brother, Scott. She attributes her life lessons of compassion for and understanding of others to Scott. E-mail her at fillingam@ec.rr.com to come and share her stories of faith with your church.

Sgt. Danger Geist was honorably discharged shortly after returning home from Afghanistan and now lives with his wife and puppy in the Chicago area. To read more of his experiences in Afghanistan visit www.burningbridge.com and pick up a copy of his book, *I am Danger; I am Prisoner.*

Marijo Herndon has developed stress management strategies that benefit the coaching programs for a leading health plan company. Her articles, ranging from humor to inspiration, appear in several publications and books. She lives in New York with her husband Dave and two rescue cats. E-mail her at marijo215@nycap.rr.com.

Laura Hollingshead has a bachelor's degree in Nursing but has held a lifelong dream of being a published author. She is currently working on a book for adult children of aging parents to assist in planning for retirement, post-retirement, and end-of-life issues.

Kimberly M. Hutmacher is the author of twenty-five books and numerous pieces of poetry, fiction, and nonfiction for magazines and anthologies. To learn more about Kimberly, her published works and her workshop offerings, please visit her website www.kimberlyhutmacher.com.

Jennie Ivey lives in Cookeville, TN. She is a newspaper columnist and the author of several works of fiction and nonfiction, including several stories in the *Chicken Soup for the Soul* series.

BJ Jensen is an author, inspirational speaker, dramatist and music-signing artist. She directs Love In Motion Signing Choir (www.signingchoir.com), which travels internationally. BJ is happily married to Dr. Doug Jensen and they live near their son, daughter-in-love, and three precious granddaughters in San Diego, CA. E-mail her at jensen2@san.rr.com.

Lynnette Jung received a B.A. degree from the College of St. Catherine in St. Paul, MN, in 1961 and her master's degree in Social Work from The University of Utah in 1965. She is retired from the USAF, and she enjoys reading, gourmet cooking, hiking and Pilates.

Nancy B. Kennedy's most recent books are the second title in her *Miracles & Moments of Grace* series, *Inspiring Stories from Doctors* (Leafwood, 2012), and *How We Did It: Weight Loss Choices That Will Work for You* (Leafwood, 2011). To learn more about her writing, visit her website at www.nancybkennedy.com.

April Knight is a freelance writer and artist. Her favorite pastime is riding horses. She also writes Christian romance novels and has a newspaper column.

Annette Langer, previous Chicken Soup for the Soul contributor, tempers occasionally-somber topics with humor. *Healing Through Humor:*

Change Your Focus, Change Your Life! chronicles her brain injury to breast cancer challenges. *A Funny Thing Happened on My Way to the World* details her travels to all seven continents. www.AnnetteLanger.com.

Phyllis McKinley recently moved from Florida to Maine without hurting her back. Her writing took triple first place awards in Florida's 2010 Royal Palm Literary Awards, in Poetry and Children's categories. She lives with her husband, Dr. Hanford Brace, in Calais, ME.

Caroline McKinney is semi-retired from the School of Education at the University of Colorado where she has been an adjunct for over twenty years. She spends time with her seven grandchildren, hiking Colorado's trails with her dog and trying to learn Italian. She enjoys writing poetry for religious publications.

Paula Naughton lives in Michigan with her husband Don, three horses, four dogs, chickens and multiple cats. She rides horses in dressage and trail. Paula enjoys raising and preserving organic food. She is a nonfiction writer and currently working on a nonfiction narrative. E-mail her at my2spottedhorses@hotmail.com.

Amy Newmark is Publisher and Editor-in-Chief of Chicken Soup for the Soul and co-authors many of the books as well. She and her husband have four grown children. You can reach Amy through webmaster@chickensoupforthesoul.com. Follow her on Twitter @amynewmark.

Jennifer Quasha is a freelance writer and editor who is the co-author of *Chicken Soup for the Soul: My Dog's Life*, *Chicken Soup for the Soul: My Cat's Life*, *Chicken Soup for the Soul: I Can't Believe My Dog Did That!* and *Chicken Soup for the Soul: I Can't Believe My Cat Did That!* Learn more at www.jenniferquasha.com.

Jennifer Reed is a children's author of over twenty-five books. She teaches Yearbook part-time and is currently working on her master's degree at Vermont College. Jennifer enjoys traveling, spending time with family and friends, and of course, writing! Visit her website at www.jennifer-reed.com.

Anna Rose Silver is a middle school student. She enjoys writing, dancing and eating pizza. Anna is the co-author of two children's books that were published by the American Cancer Society titled *Our Mom Is Getting Better* and *Our Dad Is Getting Better.*

Diane Stokes received her Bachelor of Science degree from UMass Lowell and an MBA degree from Clark University. She is a founder at Oncology Rehab Partners, a company advancing cancer and survivorship rehab, and FitBricks, a triathlon coaching company. She enjoys competing in triathlons of all distances. E-mail her at dstokes@FitBricks.com.

Samantha Ducloux Waltz is an award-winning freelance writer in Portland, OR. Her personal stories have appeared in the *Chicken Soup for the Soul* series, numerous other anthologies, *The Christian Science Monitor* and *Redbook.* She has also written fiction and nonfiction under the name Samellyn Wood. Learn more at www.pathsofthought.com.

Bill Wetterman is a retired Vice President from an executive search firm. His second career is freelance writing, and he's working on several novels. E-mail him at bwetterman@cox.net.

About the Author

Julie Silver, MD is an assistant professor at Harvard Medical School in the Department of Physical Medicine and Rehabilitation. Dr. Silver is an award-winning author and has written many books including: *You Can Heal Yourself: A Guide to Physical and Emotional Recovery After Injury or Illness*; *After Cancer Treatment: Heal Faster, Better, Stronger*; and *What Helped Get Me Through: Cancer Survivors Share Wisdom and Hope*.

Dr. Silver is the Chief Editor of Books at Harvard Health Publications, the consumer health publishing branch of Harvard Medical School. She is responsible for all of the books that officially come from Harvard Medical School. These publications include new science and cutting-edge concepts such as The Almost Effect™ series of books that describes subclinical symptoms in behavioral health and psychology. You can learn more about this at www.TheAlmostEffect.com.

She is also the co-founder of Oncology Rehab Partners which has developed the STAR Program® Certifications—a best practices and evidence-based model for oncology rehabilitation care. Her work in cancer rehabilitation has been recognized by the American Cancer Society, and she was awarded the prestigious Lane Adams Quality of Life Award. She was also chosen by Massachusetts General Hospital for THE ONE HUNDRED award that is given to 100 people in the United States who are making a significant difference in cancer care.

Dr. Silver is currently on the medical staff at Spaulding Rehabilitation, Massachusetts General and Brigham and Women's hospitals. Her work has been featured on many national media outlets including *Today*, *The Early Show*, *The Dr. Oz Show*, *ABC News Now*, AARP Radio and NPR. You can learn more about her work at www.JulieSilverMD.com and www.OncologyRehabPartners.com.

Acknowledgments

In undertaking any book on healing, my mission is always to alleviate unnecessary pain, suffering and disability. My work is firmly focused on helping people recover as well as possible using the latest science in rehabilitation medicine. I am not alone in this mission and so first I would like to acknowledge with gratitude my colleagues who are physicians specializing in Physical Medicine and Rehabilitation — physiatrists. Next, I thank the many other healthcare professionals who are dedicated to rehabilitation medicine and helping people to live optimally no matter what constitutes their underlying illness or injury.

Bringing important health information to the public is a core mission of Harvard Medical School. As the Chief Editor of Books at Harvard Health Publications, I work with many people who deserve mention. However, in an effort to be brief, those who should be recognized for this collaboration with Chicken Soup for the Soul include Rusty Shelton, Anthony Komaroff, Ed Coburn, Natalie Ramm, Robert O'Connell and Linda Konner. On the Chicken Soup for the Soul side, no one has worked harder on this series of books than Amy Newmark.

I am immensely grateful to the people who shared their stories in this collection. There were far too many wonderful contributions to use them all in this book, and we chose the ones that worked best with the medical information presented. I firmly believe that everyone's life experiences have much to teach all of us, and it is truly a privilege to have the opportunity to share these stories with readers.

Finally, I want to thank my family, especially my daughter, Anna Rose, who agreed to write a story about her experience with neck pain.

If you are in need of healing, I hope that this book provides you with some helpful strategies as well as inspiration to take with you on your journey.